Nursing Assistant

A Basic Study Guide

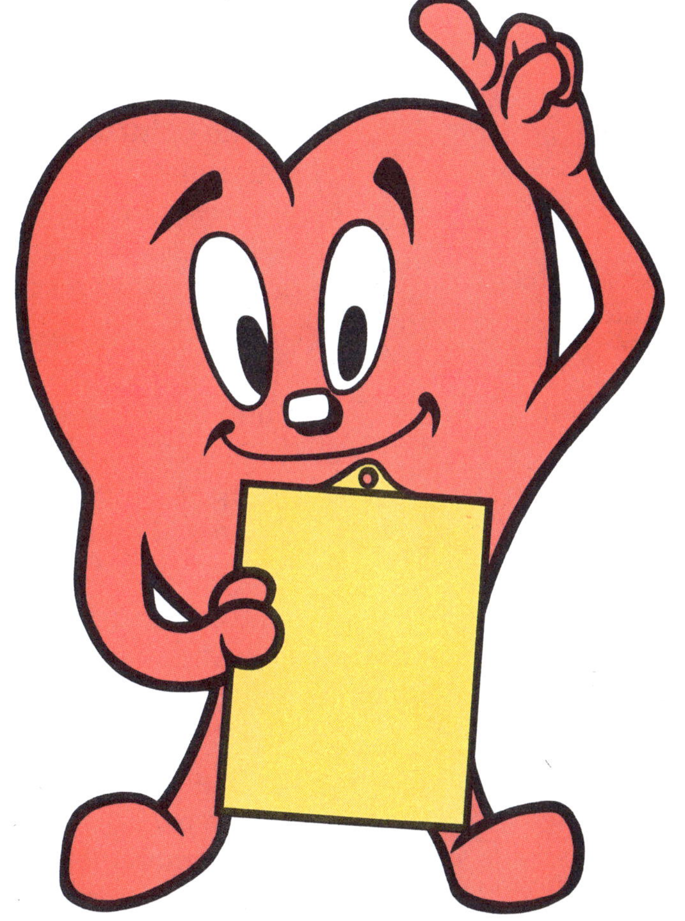

Beverly Robertson, MSC
FIRST CLASS BOOKS, INC.

Acknowledgments

With appreciation to the following for their technical advice:

Mary Ann Bruggink, LPN, CNA
St. Luke's Extended Care Facility

Elizabeth Dressel, RN, DNS
Director of Nursing
Menlo Park Health Care Center

Cheryl Hoffman, RN, BSN, ICP
Director of Education
St. Luke's Extended Care Facility

David Langdon
Administrator
Menlo Park Health Care Center

Christina Spencer, BSN RN, C
Nursing Assistant Training Institute

Alicia Steed, RN, BSN, CCRN
Sacred Heart Medical Center

Gloria Williams, MA, DSDE, LVN
Director of Training
Pioneer House

Barbara Bailey,
Production Coordinator

Special thanks to Jackie for her wisdom and caring, and to many other public officials who must remain anonymous.

About the Author. . .

Beverly Robertson has worked with adult education since 1974, developing classes, recruiting and training teachers, and observing and evaluating teaching methods. Beverly earned a master's degree in communications in 1990. Her adult education experiences and communications skills are evident in this easy-to-read, easy-to-understand study guide.

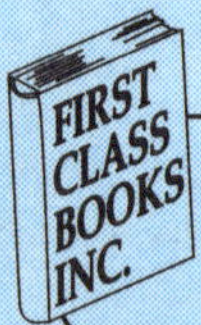

6012 E. Broadway
Spokane, Washington 99212
1-800-524-9911

Welcome. . .

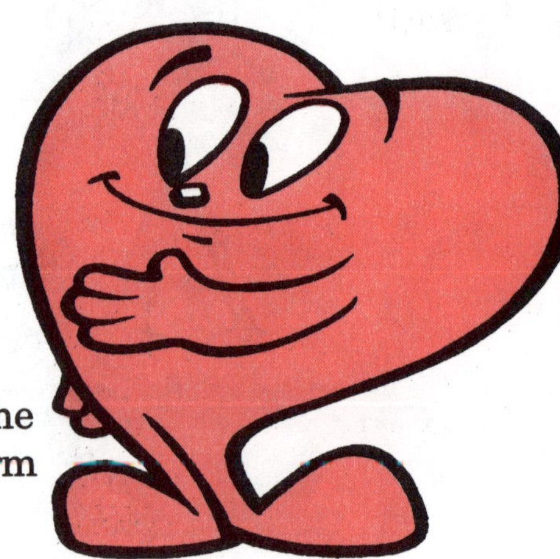

. . .to the honorable career of Nursing Assistant. You have made a wise career choice that provides professional skills in the rapidly growing area of long-term health care.

How to Use this Book

Each **Lesson** outlines several **Objectives** so you will know the points to look for in the text. Read the lesson until you understand each **Part**. Then check your knowledge by answering the questions in the **NA Review** at the end of each lesson. Write class notes on the **NA Notes** pages to remind you of important points.

To help you understand the terminology that you will use in your new job, there are **Key Words** with pronunciation and meaning at the end of each lesson and a **Glossary** at the back of the book. The **Tips and Terms** study cards will help you learn medical abbreviations and recognize symptoms of potential medical problems. Cut out the cards and start using them right away.

The **Appendix** lists **Practical Skills** that the NA practices during clinical training. You will also find **Medical Abbreviations** to assist you in reading the patients' charts.

The **Heart "Care"acter** that illustrates the book represents the caring heart that is so vital in the nursing profession. The more you read, write, and review the material in this book, the more quickly you will learn it. Your new skills, along with your caring attitude, will earn the friendship and trust of your patients, the respect of your employer and co-workers, and personal satisfaction.

Contents

Cut-out *Tips and Terms Flashcards*
at back of book

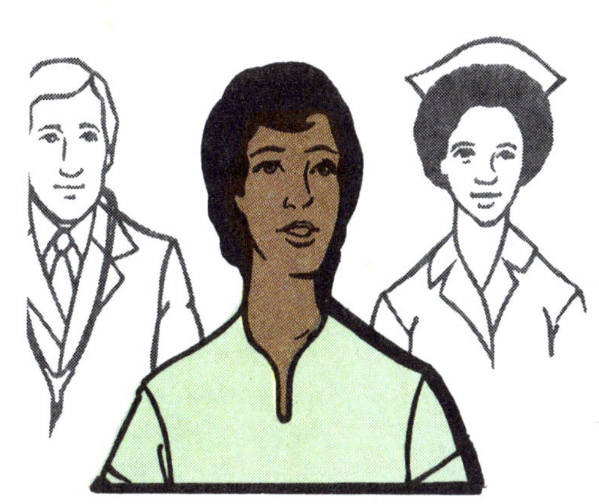

The Nursing Assistant (NA)

The Nursing Assistant (NA) spends more time with the patient than any other member of the health-care team!

Objectives:

- ☐ Identify the duties and concerns of the NA
- ☐ Discuss the importance of the health-care team
- ☐ Explain patient rights
- ☐ Identify legal issues

<table><tr><td>**Part 1**</td><td># Being Professional</td></tr></table>

Your patients and your employer depend on you.

Earn the trust of your patients and your employer by being the most professional NA you can be. Set high standards for yourself.

Confidentiality

Information about patients is very private. You have both a legal and moral responsibility to keep patient information confidential.

Dedication

No task is unimportant if it contributes to the patient's well-being.

Honesty

Complete all assignments. Do not skip tasks or chart records until the task is completed.

Respect the patient's personal possessions; there may be legal action if possessions are lost.

Integrity

Perform duties to the best of your ability. If in doubt, request clear instructions. Know and follow the employer's work rules. Follow the Patient Bill of Rights (see page 8).

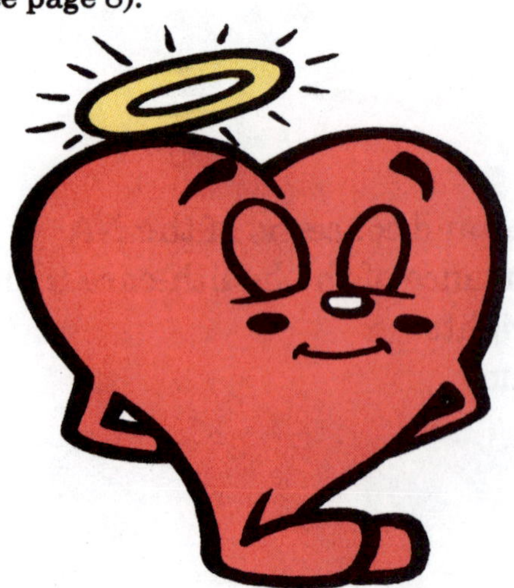

Loyalty

Support the ideals of the health-care facility.

Reliability

Patients and staff must be able to depend on you. Be on time for work, in proper uniform and well-groomed. If you are unable to work, notify your supervisor at least two hours before your shift begins.

Observe and chart information accurately. Notify your supervisor promptly of problems or changes in the patient's condition.

Respect

Always show respect for patients, families, and staff members (even if you dislike them).

Unacceptable Behaviors

Unacceptable behavior may result in dismissal!

Never use verbal or physical abuse.

Do not steal or willfully damage property.

Never disobey an order from a supervisor.

Do not neglect your duties.

Never alter or falsify any records or reports.

Do not work under the influence of drugs or alcohol.

Do not lie.

Part 2 — Keeping the Whole Person Healthy

The NA is an important member of the health-care team.

A health-care team provides total care for each patient. The NA is an important member of the health-care team and spends more time with the patient than any other member. The NA's attitude and skills affect the patient's behavior and well-being.

It is important for the NA to understand the facility's administrative structure and proper reporting procedures.

The Health-care Team

The most important member of the health-care team is the patient. The patient should have a say in personal care and should always be encouraged to be as independent as possible.

Other members of the health-care team are the nursing staff, doctors, therapists, dietitians, administration, activity staff, and family.

Care Plans

The health-care team develops individual care plans for each patient. Carrying out the plan is a team effort. Check the care plan for each patient and carry out instructions carefully. Total health care is everything that contributes to the patient's wellness:

- proper medical attention
- balanced diet
- exercise
- rest and comfort
- emotional, social, and spiritual well-being

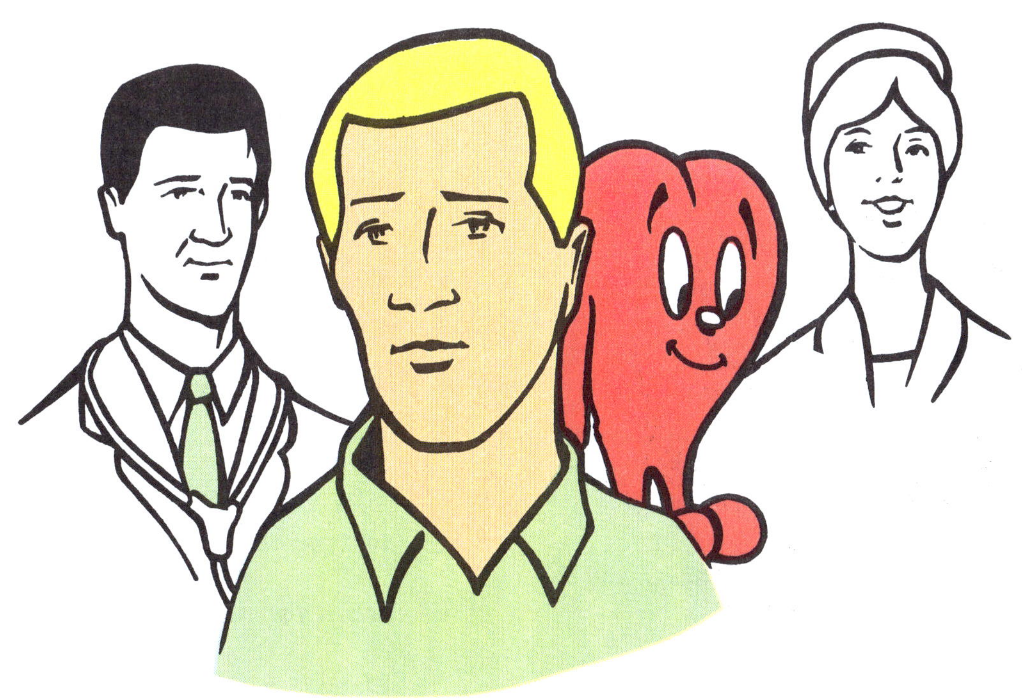

Part 3 — Respecting the Patient's Rights

The NA has a legal responsibility to protect patient rights.

The **Patient's Bill of Rights** is a legal document that protects the residents in health-care facilities.

Patient Rights

The bill assures each patient:

- free choice

- the right to complete information about health and treatment

- participation in planning medical treatment

- considerate and respectful care

- the right to refuse treatment

- freedom from physical or mental abuse

- freedom from discrimination

- privacy and confidentiality

- the right to keep and use personal belongings

- the right to send and receive unopened mail

- choice of religious activities

- assistance in filing complaints

- participation in resident and family groups

- the right to examine survey results

- management and security of personal funds

- information about services and charges

- advance notice of transfer or discharge and the right to appeal

- safe and orderly transfer or discharge

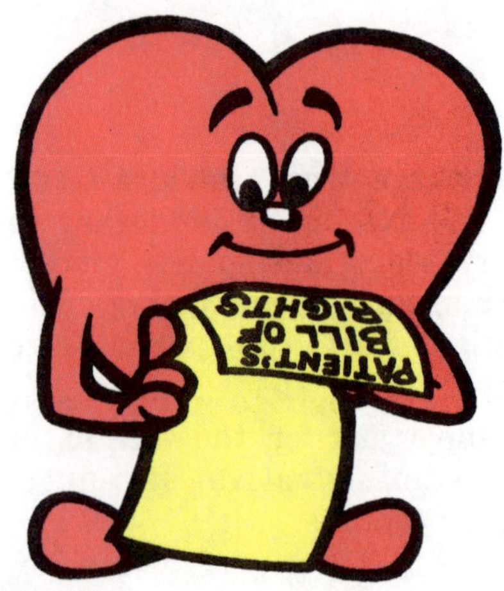

Legal Issues

It is your legal responsibility to respect the patients' rights and to protect them from physical or mental harm. Legal action may result from abuse or failure to report suspected abuse. If a patient has a complaint, report it.

- **Elder abuse**: Physical, sexual, medical, or psychological abuse; exploitation and neglect.

- **Abuse**: Mental, physical, or financial abuse, or the failure to report suspected abuse.

- **Assault**: Threat of bodily harm.

- **Battery**: Carrying out a threat.

- **False Documentation**: Entries in a patient's record that are not true or have been altered.

- **Negligence**: Failure to give assigned care, or giving improper care that causes harm.

  Example: failure to raise bedrails and the patient falls from the bed.

- **Defamation**: Falsehoods that result in damage to a person's reputation or character.

  Libel: a written statement.

  Slander: a spoken statement.

<table><tr><td>Part 4</td><td>

Respecting the Patient's Beliefs

</td></tr></table>

The NA should encourage the patient to continue religious practices, whatever they may be.

Whatever a patient's approach to the meaning of life, it is the NA's responsibility to respect the patient's beliefs.

- Be sensitive to the patient.

- Support the right to practice individual beliefs.

- Make sure your speech and actions do not offend others.

- Be respectful of the patient's customs and possessions.

- Show interest in the beliefs of your patients.

- Be willing to listen if they wish to talk.

- Never question or make fun of another's beliefs.

- Never try to force your religious beliefs on a patient.

A patient does not have to be a member of an organized religion to have spiritual needs. Spiritual needs can be expressed by a way of life or through everyday activities.

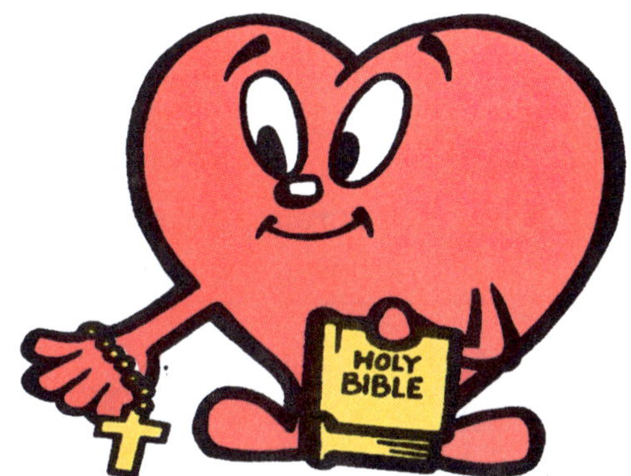

A patient may have religious items in the room (such as rosaries or prayer books). The NA should respect these items. If you must move them, handle them with respect.

Religious Customs

Learn about a patient's religious customs. The more you know, the less likely you are to accidently offend someone.

Holidays

Be aware of days celebrated with special rituals. The patient may need extra help dressing for a special holiday or may need privacy for a certain ritual (such as confession for Catholics).

Foods

Some religions forbid certain foods. Know what is not allowed and offer other choices. Determine special times the patient may want to fast (go without food) or eat only certain foods.

Clothing

Some religions (such as Jewish, Mormon) have certain articles of clothing. Treat these with respect.

Medical Treatments

Be aware of any medical treatments that are not allowed (such as blood transfusions for Jehovah's Witnesses).

Clergy

When clergy members visit patients, ensure privacy if desired. When a patient wants to see a clergy member, make sure your supervisor is informed.

NA Review

1. Explain why confidentiality is important.

____

____

____

____

2. Choose one area of professionalism and describe why you feel it is important.

____

____

____

____

____

3. Identify behaviors that result in dismissal.

____

____

____

____

____

____

4. Who is the health-care team?

____

____

____

____

5. What is total care?

____

____

____

____

6. Identify six or more patient rights.

1.) Confidentiality

____

____

____

____

7. Describe legal issues related to patient care.

____

____

____

____

Vocabulary

Note on Pronunciation: The vocabulary that follows each lesson will help you with the key words. Become familiar with the words by saying them aloud. The correct spelling is followed by phonetic spelling to help you pronounce each word, one syllable at a time, with bold print for emphasis.

assault	(ah-**sawlt**)	threat of bodily harm
battery	(**bat**-er-ree)	physical attack or harm
confidentiality	(kon-fi-den-che-**al**-i-tee)	not revealing private information about others
defamation	(de-fuh-**may**-shun)	oral or written words that damage someone's reputation
false documentation	(fawls dock-yu-men-**tay**-shun)	knowingly putting incorrect information on a patient's record
negligence	(**neg**-li-jens)	careless patient care

Additional Terms to Remember

____

____

____

____

____

____

____

____

____

____

____

Many English words and letters can be pronounced in different ways. This is the most common pronunciation, following the system used in Blakison's *Gould Medical Dictionary*, 4th edition. In some cases questions were settled by referring to Dorland's *Illustrated Medical Dictionary*, 26th edition, which closely follows Gould. For nonmedical terms, the *Dictionary of Pronunciation*, 2nd edition, by Samuel Noory, was used, but spellings of word sounds are consistent with Gould.

NA Notes

The most important member of the health-care team is the patient!

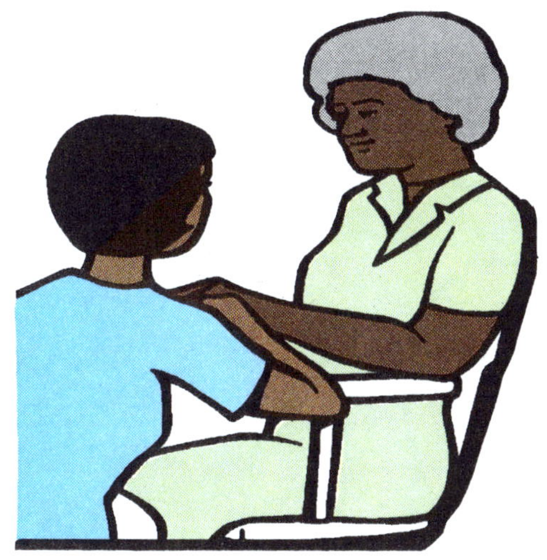

Relating to your Patients

Everything you do or say communicates a message!

Objectives:

- ☐ Identify basic needs
- ☐ Demonstrate ways to develop positive relationships
- ☐ Recognize the patient's concerns
- ☐ Use effective communication skills

Part 1 — Understanding Basic Needs

Help your patients feel good about themselves and reach for their dreams.

The famous psychologist, Abraham Maslow, identified steps for meeting needs in his Hierarchy of Human Needs. A person's needs must be satisfied at one level before moving upward in a step-by-step progression from basic physical needs toward self-actualization. The NA plays an important role in meeting the patient's needs.

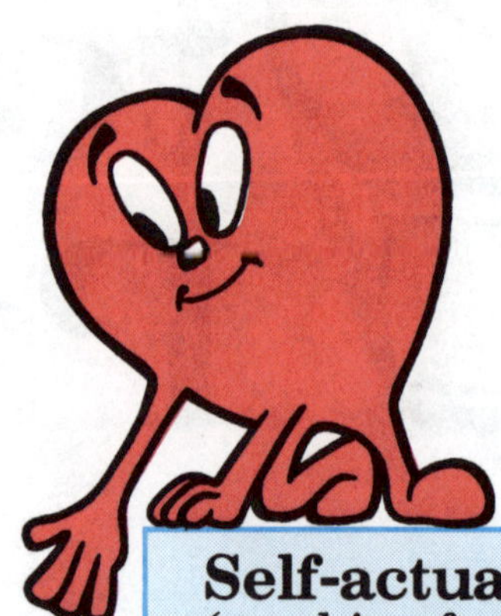

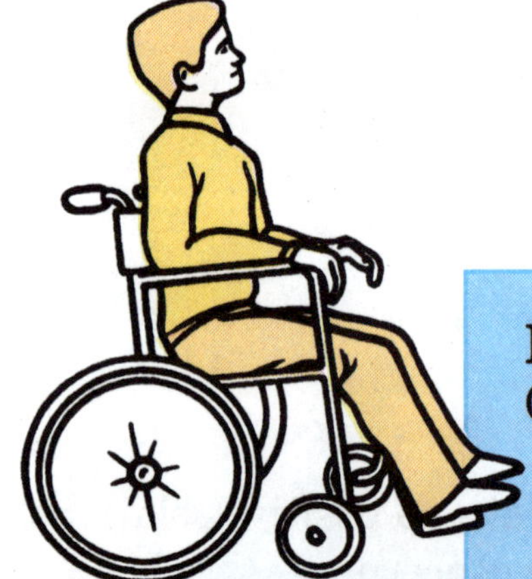

Self-actualization
(reaching for dreams)

- Be enthusiastic and supportive.
- Encourage projects and plans.
- Be positive about the future.
- Promote optimism.

Self-esteem
(pride)

- Encourage independence.
- Praise when appropriate.
- Welcome ideas and suggestions.
- Respect beliefs and belongings.
- Be supportive.
- Treat the patient with dignity.

Belonging
(feeling accepted)

- Show that you care.
- Promote interaction with others.
- Listen attentively.
- Be patient.
- Make the patient feel "at home."
- Show respect for family and friends.

Safety and Security
(safe from harm)

- Provide safe surroundings.
- Be alert to potential hazards.
- Know the facility's emergency procedures.
- Respond to call lights quickly.
- Maintain confidentiality.
- Provide privacy as desired.
- Observe/chart accurate information.
- Report problems.

Physical
(survival requirements)

- Deliver food trays.
- Supply fresh water.
- Assist with eating and encourage fluids.
- Assist with elimination as needed.
- Position for comfort and easy breathing.

Building Relationships

*Treating your patients with respect and
dignity builds good relationships.*

Good relationships are the foundation for a comfortable working experience.

Basic Guidelines

Always knock before entering a patient's room. Remember that this is the patient's living quarters. Provide the privacy and courtesy you would show to people in their own homes.

Introduce yourself. Some patients have difficulty remembering names. Say your name whenever you enter to avoid confusion or embarrassment for the patient.

Ask how the patient wishes to be addressed. Many elderly patients do not wish to be called by their first names.

Offer choices. Whenever possible, offer the patient choices. For example, your schedule may permit you to give the patient a bath now or in 30 minutes. Offer the patient a choice. Choices encourage independence. Be specific in your options. Stick to your promises, or let the patient know if you will be late.

Provide comfort. Pay attention to the patient's needs. Provide adequate ventilation, warmth, light, and quiet.

Be courteous and respectful of visitors. Family and friends influence the patient's well-being. Provide privacy if desired. If you must give care, politely ask visitors to leave the room, and let them know when they can return.

Maintain privacy and dignity at all times. Everyone wants to be loved and have friends with shared interests. Regardless of age, people are sexual beings with sexual thoughts and desires. The NA must deal with **sexuality** in a mature, professional manner. Allow patients plenty of privacy, and do not interfere with consenting partners as long as no one is in danger of physical harm. If problems arise, ask your supervisor how to handle the situation.

Unexpected Behaviors

Recognizing the link between actions and needs helps build good relationships. Keep in mind that long-term-care patients are adjusting to changes in their life-styles that affect them physically, emotionally, and socially.

Sometimes patients are uncooperative, demanding, threatening, rude, or stubborn. Try to look beyond the behavior to the underlying need for comfort and understanding.

Some concerns that affect the patient's behavior:

- anxiety
- loneliness
- health concerns
- pain
- change in life-style
- loss of independence
- unmet expectations
- fear
- grief
- financial concerns
- longing for the "old days"
- lack of understanding
- unmet physical and social needs
- religious concerns
- family problems
- depression
- lack of self-esteem
- physical and mental problems
- sleeplessness

Always respond with patience, caring, **empathy** (sharing another's emotion), concern, and kindness. The patient's well-being is your primary concern. If the problem continues, ask your supervisor for help.

Part 3 — Using Good Communication Skills

The way you treat patients affects their behavior.

NAs need good communication skills. The ability to communicate well builds good working relations with patients and the health-care team.

Speaking, listening, feedback, and actions are important for everything you do:

- provide proper care
- show concern for patients
- get along with patients, families, and co-workers
- reduce conflict
- report observations
- give directions
- follow directions
- learn by listening
- send accurate messages
- explain procedures
- define problems

Communication simply means sending and receiving messages. However, effective communication involves more than words. Both verbal and nonverbal messages carry meaning. Always treat the patients with respect.

Verbal: *Words, spoken or written.* Use simple and clear words.

Nonverbal: *Body language.* Everything you do sends a message:

- facial expression
- gestures
- tone of voice
- posture
- eye contact
- silence
- touch

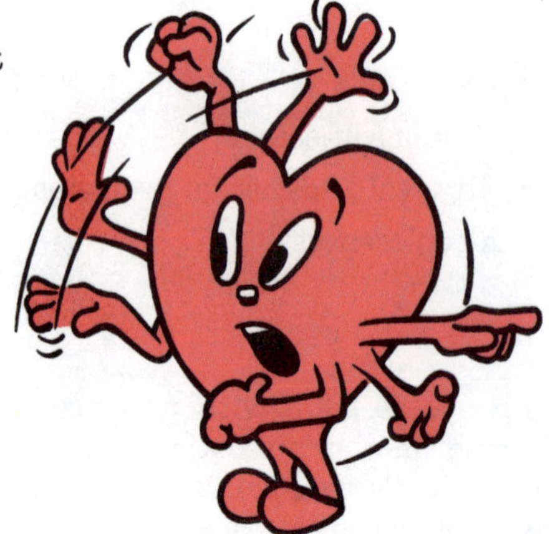

Verbal and nonverbal language must agree in order to send clear messages.

The problem is that most people are not aware of their nonverbal behavior. Unless verbal and nonverbal language agree, the listener gets a mixed message. For example, if the NA expresses caring and concern, but stands with folded arms and a look of disgust, the patient gets conflicting messages. Unfortunately, when messages are mixed, the nonverbal impressions speak louder than the words.

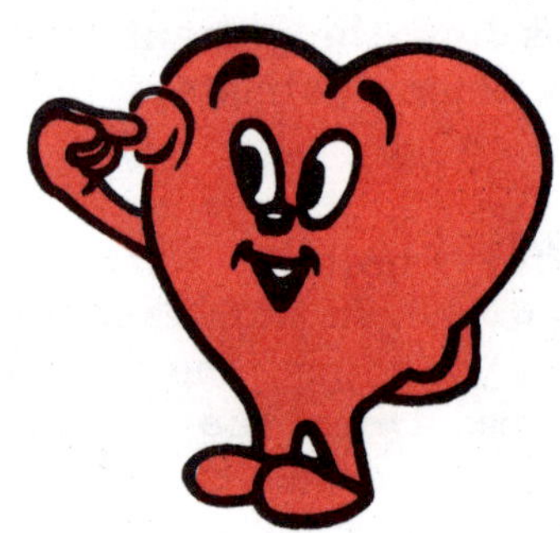

Listening

Pay attention to what the other person is saying. Listen for facts and listen for feelings. Ask questions when you don't understand.

By being a good listener, the NA can learn what the patient likes and doesn't like, as well as problems, concerns, interests, and needs.

Feedback

Words have different meanings to different people, which can lead to misunderstandings. To be sure that you understand what others say to you, **paraphrase** (repeat what you heard using your own words). Ask if the statement is correct.

Check whether others understand what you are saying by asking questions and encouraging feedback.

Guidelines for Effective Communication

- Be patient.
- Be a good listener.
- Use short sentences.
- Avoid criticizing.
- Be aware of body language.
- Show interest.
- Use a friendly tone.
- Be positive.
- Use eye contact.
- Speak clearly.
- Ask for feedback.
- Clarify as needed.
- Use words the person understands.
- Show respect.
- Pace yourself.

Barriers to Good Communication

- patronizing
- threatening
- preaching
- using harsh language
- interrupting
- being a know-it-all
- misunderstandings
- arguing
- ordering
- belittling
- ignoring
- changing the subject
- being too busy
- cultural differences

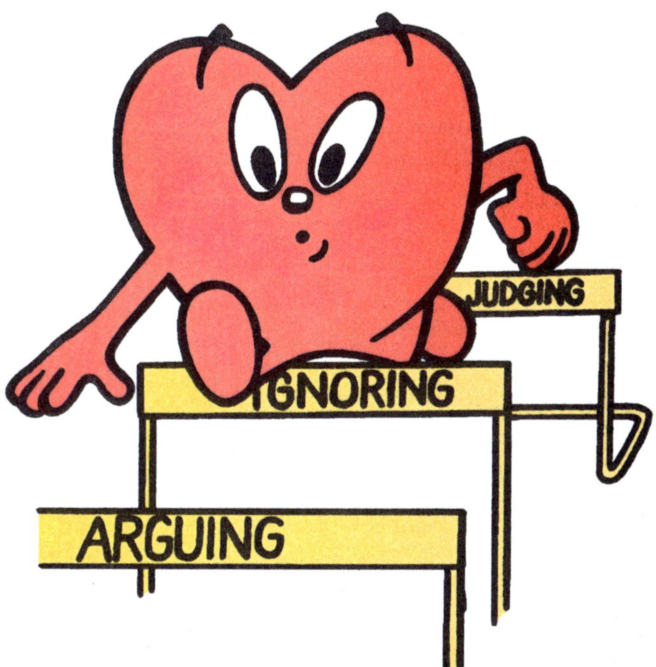

Part 4 Communicating with the Sensory Impaired

Improve your communication with people who have difficulty seeing or hearing by remembering a few basic guidelines.

Hearing Impaired

To communicate with people who have hearing problems:

- Get close to the person and speak loudly enough to be heard without shouting.
- Speak to the side where hearing is best.
- Maintain eye contact.
- Ask for feedback to determine understanding.
- Eliminate unnecessary noises. (For example, turn off the T.V. or radio.)
- If the patient uses a hearing aid, make sure he or she is wearing it. Be sure it is clean.
- Make sure you face the patient who reads lips.
- Use gestures.

Visually Impaired

To communicate with people who have vision problems:

- Identify yourself when entering the room.
- Explain what you are going to do.
- Ask for feedback.
- Remind the patient to wear glasses if needed, and offer to help clean the glasses.

NA Review

1. Why is it important for the NA to understand basic needs?

____

____

____

____

____

2. Identify five or more ways to build positive relationships with patients.

1.) Offer choices whenever possible.

____

____

____

____

3. Why should you knock before entering the patient's room?

____

____

____

____

4. What is the connection between concerns and behavior?

____

____

____

5. Why does the NA need good communication skills?

____

____

____

____

6. Describe nonverbal communication.

____

____

____

____

7. Why is feedback important?

____

____

____

____

Vocabulary

barrier	(**ba**-ree-er)	obstacle blocking approach, path or goal
feedback	(**feed**-back)	repeat message to confirm understanding
nonverbal	(**non**-ver-bal)	body language, facial expressions, hand gestures
paraphrase	(**pa**-ra-fraze)	repeating statement in your own words
self-actualization	(self-ack-chew-al-i-**zay**-shun)	achieving dreams or goals

Additional Terms to Remember

NA Notes

My attitude affects the patient's attitude.

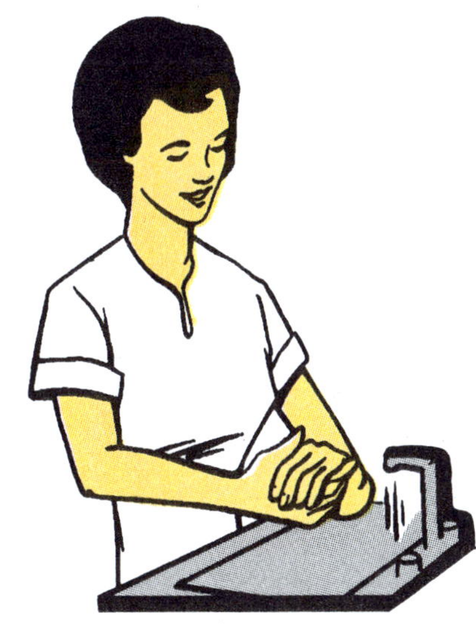

Infection Control

Wash your hands before and after every contact with patients or equipment!

Objectives:

- ☐ Discuss Universal Precautions
- ☐ Explain how to control HBV
- ☐ Identify ways that AIDS is transmitted
- ☐ Describe ways to prevent infection
- ☐ Explain procedures for sterilizing and disinfecting
- ☐ Describe isolation procedures
- ☐ Demonstrate proper handwashing
- ☐ Identify protective barriers

<table><tr><td>Part 1</td><td></td></tr></table>

Precautions

Protect against possible infection at all times.

Infection control is a major concern for health-care workers. Universal precautions (UP) were developed in 1988 to prevent the spread of deadly blood-borne viruses and bacteria.

Universal precautions establish safe practices for health-care workers to control the spread of Acquired Immune Deficiency Syndrome (AIDS) and Hepatitis B virus (HBV). Because health-care workers do not know who is infected, the precautions apply to all patients.

Universal Precautions

Universal precautions apply to all patients, all used needles, and all body fluids. Assume all blood, body fluids, and needles are potentially infectious. Gloves must be worn at all times when handling these materials to avoid infection.

Infected people often have no symptoms and may not know they are infected. Therefore, consider yourself at risk of infection from all patients.

Feces (body waste), urine, sweat, vomit, or nose and mouth secretions are sources of **cross-contamination** (passed from one person to another).

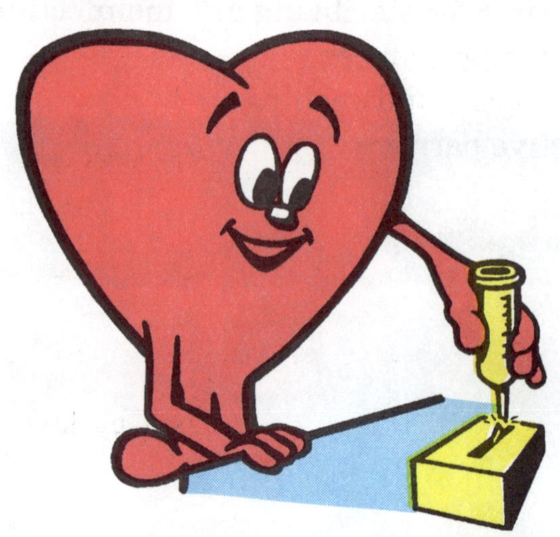

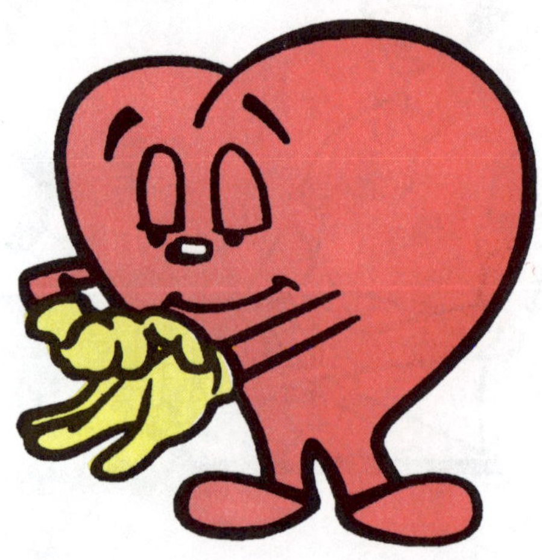

Gloves

Always inspect gloves before use. Do not use gloves that are torn or cracked, have holes, or are faded.

Always wear gloves when:

- handling blood or body fluids.
- tending persons with bed sores, broken skin, rashes, or bleeding.
- handling linens soiled with blood or other body fluids.
- cleaning up spills containing blood or body fluids.

Needles

All health-care professionals who handle needles must use extra caution.

- Be aware that the gloves will not protect you from needlesticks.
- Dispose of needles in proper disposal containers.

Other Precautions

- If you are pregnant and working in a high-risk area, get medical counseling.
- Report all broken skin contact, mucous membrane contact, and puncture wounds.
- Wash hands after disposing of gloves.

Controlling Hepatitis B Virus (HBV)

Vaccination can prevent HBV infection.

HBV is a viral infection of the liver. It produces fatigue, mild fever, muscle and joint pain, nausea, vomiting, and loss of appetite.

There is no known cure for HBV. A blood test is the only way to find out if you are infected. Get a blood test; if you are not infected, be vaccinated to prevent infection.

HBV usually spreads through contact with infected blood, blood products, and bodily fluids. However, the virus can be found in urine, feces, semen, tears, saliva, vaginal fluid, and breast milk.

The virus is transmitted primarily through:

- intimate sexual contact.
- puncture wounds from contaminated needles or sharp objects.
- mucous membranes (eyes, nose, or mouth).
- damaged skin (cuts, rashes, dry skin).

Be tested for HBV. If you test negative, get vaccinated!

Preventing AIDS

Health-care workers must take special precautions with body fluids, especially blood.

AIDS is caused by the virus **HIV** (human immunodeficiency virus). AIDS cripples the **immune system** (the body's natural defense against disease), and the person eventually dies from infections.

AIDS kills! There is no cure! Protect yourself and your patients from infection.

When people are infected with HIV, they **are** carriers for life. Some carriers never show symptoms, but can still **transmit** (pass on) HIV to others.

Some people develop mild symptoms of the disease a few days after infection:

- flu-like sickness
- swollen glands
- rash
- fever

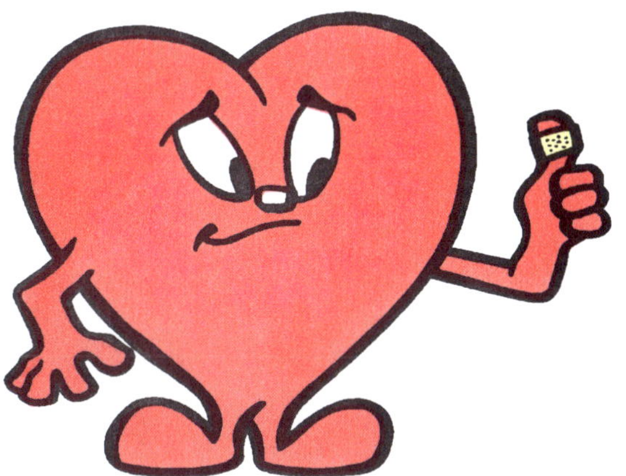

These symptoms go away, but the HIV remains in the body. There is no cure and no vaccine for HIV. Advanced symptoms may develop five to fourteen years later.

The disease is transmitted when **contaminated** (infected) fluid enters the bloodstream.

Ways HIV is transmitted:

- blood
- body fluids that contain blood
- semen
- vaginal secretions

Of these, blood is the most common concern for the health-care worker.

Ways HIV enters the body:

- puncture wounds from infected needles or broken glass
- cuts or open sores
- mucous membranes (nose, mouth, eyes)
- intimate sexual contact
- transfusions with infected blood
- infected hypodermic needles
- infected mothers to their unborn babies

<table><tr><td>Part 4</td><td>

Preventing Infection
</td></tr></table>

Preventing problems is better than curing mistakes.

Infection control is critical! By understanding how infection spreads, NAs can protect themselves and their patients.

Three steps for controlling infection:

- protect all persons from infection by others
- prevent reinfection while recuperating
- provide surroundings free of disease-causing germs

Infection is spread by **microorganisms** (living germs that can be seen only with a microscope).

Microorganisms are everywhere — in the air, on the skin, in food and beverages, and on everything you touch.

There are two types of microorganisms:

- **non-pathogenic** (harmless)
- **pathogenic** (harmful)

Pathogens are spread in five ways:

- through the air
- direct personal contact (touching the person)
- indirect contact (touching contaminated objects)
- through food, water, or blood
- from people, animals, or insects (sneezing, coughing, touching animals)

Microorganisms that cause disease are:

- **bacteria**
     staphylococci (staph)
     streptococcus (strept)
- **virus**
- **fungus**

Always report signs of infection:

• fever	• chills	• restlessness
• swelling	• redness	• lack of appetite
• pain	• discharge	• change in behavior

Infection usually enters the body through broken or damaged skin, or through the mucous membranes of the eyes, nose, or mouth.

Keeping Surroundings Clean

Help control infection with clean surroundings. Keeping the surroundings clean includes cold sterilization, disinfection, proper linen handling, and isolation.

Sterilization

Sterilizing kills all bacteria. Unless **all** bacteria are dead, an object is not sterile. A sterile object becomes contaminated when exposed to air or other objects. Diagnostic equipment and metal bedpans are most commonly sterilized by **autoclaving** (an intense heat process).

Disinfecting

Disinfecting requires chemicals that kill most of the bacteria. Those that are not killed are slowed in their growth. Reusable plastic bed pans, trays, and equipment are **sanitized** (washed in a bacterial cleanser), dried, and stored in clean paper bags.

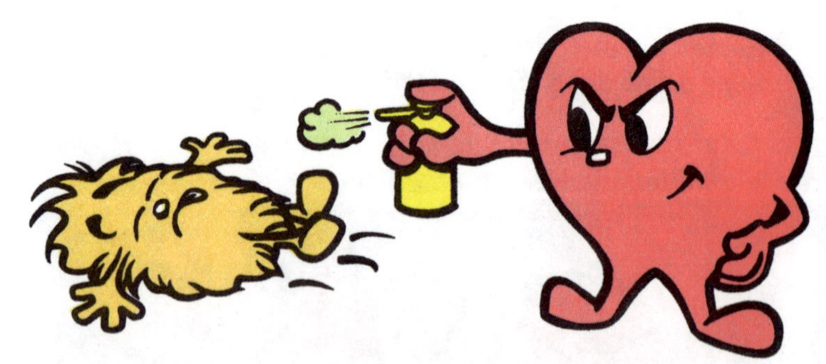

Linen Handling

- Hold linens away from you to prevent transferring microorganisms.
- Avoid shaking or fluffing linens.
- Wear gloves to handle linens that are soiled with blood or body fluids.
- Place soiled linens in covered hampers or bags to prevent the spread of infection and control odors.
- Always wash your hands after handling soiled linens.

Isolation

Isolation (setting apart) procedures are used when extra precautions are necessary to control the spread of infection.

People with contagious diseases are sometimes isolated to protect both the patients and the staff from infection. Isolation may be ordered for a patient who cannot fight infection because of age, illness, or medications. Doctors order isolation precautions, which vary according to the specific problem. It is very important to follow the doctor's orders.

Signs are posted on the door requiring visitors to report to the nursing station before entering. Depending on the type of infection, surgical gowns, gloves, and masks may be required.

All basic supplies and equipment for the care of the isolated patient should be stored in the room. Gather any additional equipment before you put on a gown and enter the room.

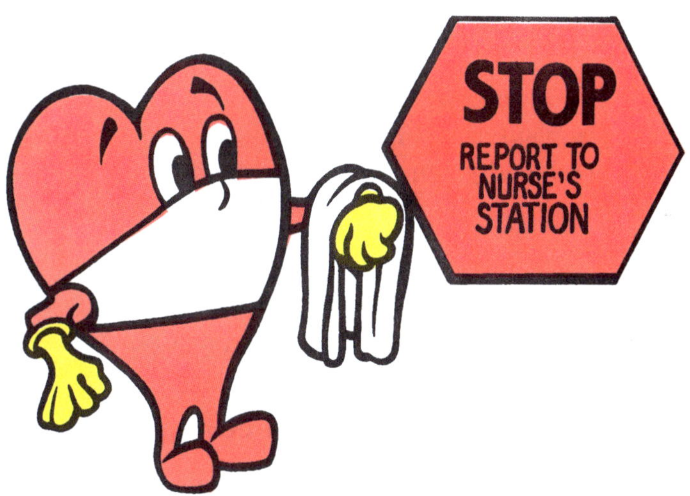

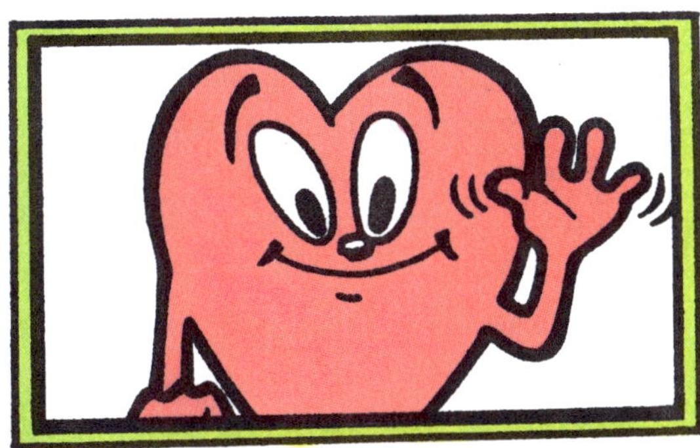

It is not uncommon for the isolated patient to be depressed. The NA can help ease depression in a variety of ways:

- Answer the call light promptly.
- Care for the isolated patient first.
- Tell the patient when you will be back; be prompt or let the patient know if you are delayed.
- Be cautious of what you say outside the room; the patient may hear you.
- Help the patient, family, and visitors be comfortable and confident with the isolation procedures.
- Provide puzzles or other amusements.
- Stop by to wave through the window.

<table>
<tr><td>Part 5</td><td><h1>Washing your Hands</h1></td></tr>
</table>

Handwashing is the most important preventive measure for infection control.

The spread of infection is greatly reduced by medical **asepsis** (procedures to decrease pathogens).

Some ways to reduce pathogens:

- hand washing
- clean surroundings
- personal hygiene

Wash your hands:

- **before and after your work shift.**
- **before and after meals.**
- **before and after patient contact.**
- **after using the toilet.**
- **after coughing, sneezing, or blowing your nose.**
- **after handling bedpans, feces, or specimens.**
- **after handling soiled linens.**

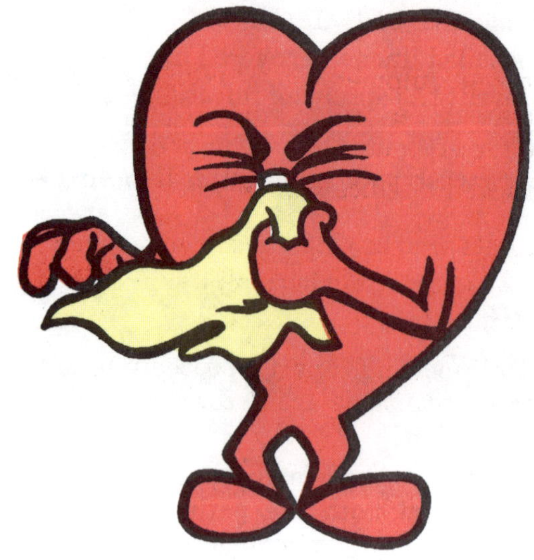

Procedure

1. Assemble equipment:
   - soap
   - paper towels
   - warm running water
   - waste basket
2. Completely wet your hands and wrists.
3. Apply soap.
4. Lather, keeping hands lower than your elbows.
5. Be sure to get soap between your fingers and under your nails.
6. Rub hands vigorously for a full minute.
7. Rinse well with running water.
8. Dry thoroughly with a paper towel.
9. Dispose of the paper towel.
10. Use a clean, dry paper towel to turn off the water.
11. Throw the paper towel away.
12. Do not touch the sink, wastebasket, or faucets with your clean hands or clothing.
13. Use hand lotion to prevent chapping from frequent hand washing.

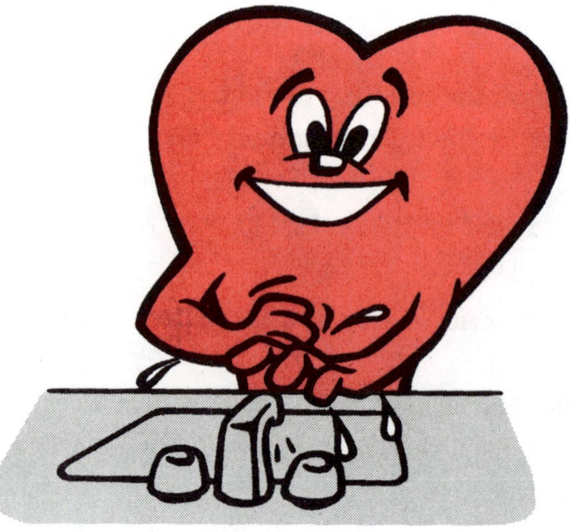

Part 6	**Using Protective Barriers**

*Always wear protective equipment as a barrier between
you and the sources of infection.*

Protective Equipment

Protective equipment such as masks, gloves, and
gowns should be worn whenever you have the
potential for exposure to blood or body fluids.

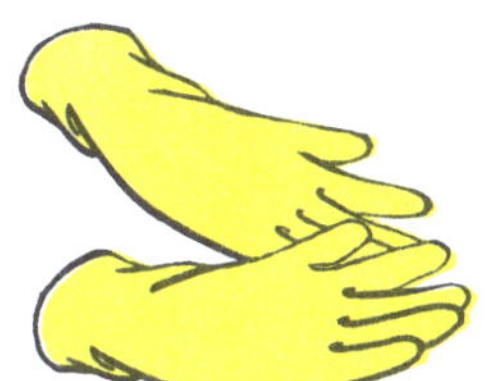

Always wear medical gloves when you contact:

- patients who are bleeding or have open
  wounds (including bedsores, skin rashes,
  or broken skin).
- blood or other body fluids.
- soiled linens.

Putting on Gloves

- Check for cracks, punctures, tears or
  discoloration.
- Discard if damaged.
- Check for proper fit.
- Pull the gloves over gown cuffs if a
  gown is worn.

Removing Gloves

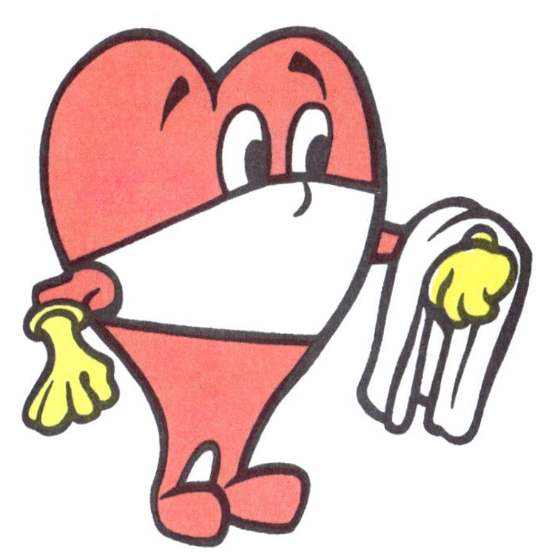

- Hold at the cuff and pull inside out.
- Fold the second glove off the hand over the
  first glove, enclosing the first glove within
  the second.
- Dispose of gloves following each patient
  contact.
- Wash your hands.

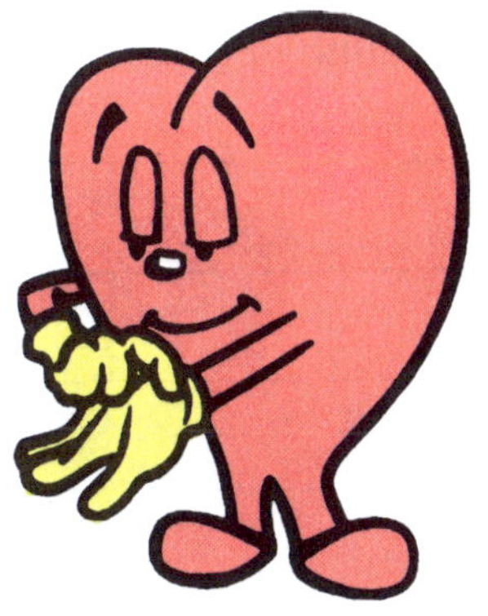

1. How do Universal Precautions (UP) apply to health-care workers?

2. How can you protect yourself from HBV?

3. Identify three or more ways that HIV infection is spread.

   1.) Puncture wounds from infected needles.

4. What is the difference between sterilizing and disinfecting?

5. Explain proper handwashing procedures and when to wash your hands.

6. Identify protective barriers and when to use them.

7. Explain isolation procedures.

Vocabulary

asepsis	(a-**sep**-sis)	procedures to reduce disease-causing organisms
autoclave	(**aw**-to-klave)	intense heat sterilizing
bacteria	(back-**te**-ree-ah)	germs causing disease that are not virus or fungus
contamination	(kon-tam-i-**nay**-shun)	to infect by contact
disinfection	(dis-in-**feck**-shun)	killing most germs or pathogens
isolation	(eye-so-**la**-shun)	separating an infected patient from others
microorganism	(my-kro-**or**-gun-iz-um)	disease-causing bacteria, virus, or fungus
pathogenic	(path-uh-**jen**-ick)	harmful germs
sterilization	(ster-i-ly-**za**-shun)	killing all microorganisms

Additional Terms to Remember

NA Notes

Washing my hands properly helps prevent the spread of germs.

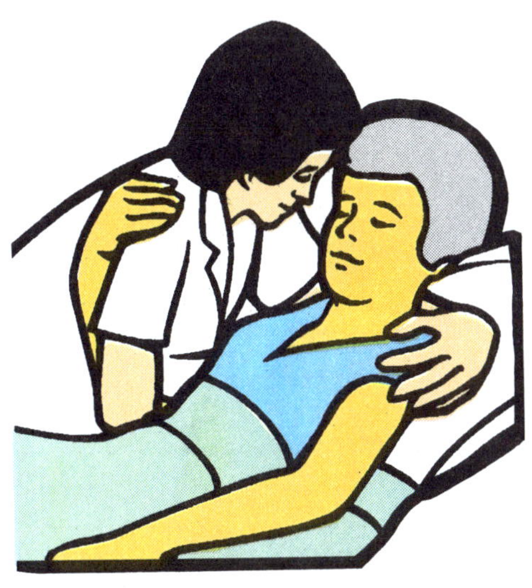

Body Mechanics

Protect the patient and yourself from injury!

Objectives:

- ☐ Demonstrate good body mechanics
- ☐ Use proper lifting techniques
- ☐ Explain the importance of positioning
- ☐ Demonstrate how to move a patient in bed
- ☐ Demonstrate how to transfer patients

Part 1	Lifting

Proper body mechanics prevent stress and injury to the patient and you.

Some patients cannot or should not move themselves. Moving patients is a major cause of accidents and injuries in the health-care profession. Using good body mechanics helps protect both you and the patient from injury.

Body mechanics are how you stand, move, and position your body. Positioning your body — back, hips, and feet — in a straight line will prevent injury, and you will not tire as easily.

Lifting Guidelines

- Evaluate the situation.
- Get help if needed.
- Lift only when necessary; push or pull whenever possible.
- Keep your back straight.
- Position your feet shoulder width apart.
- Bend your knees and lift with your leg muscles.

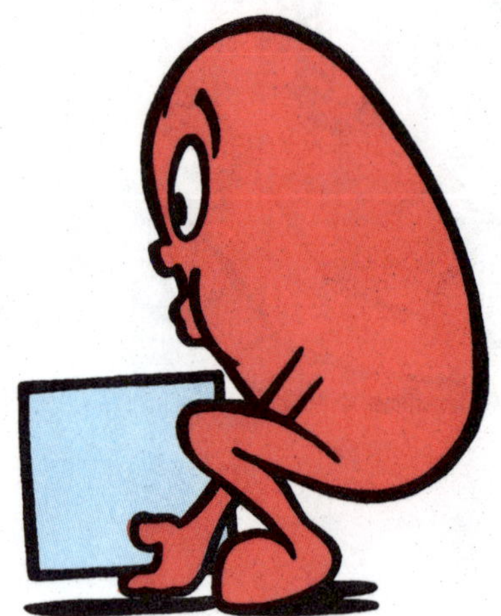

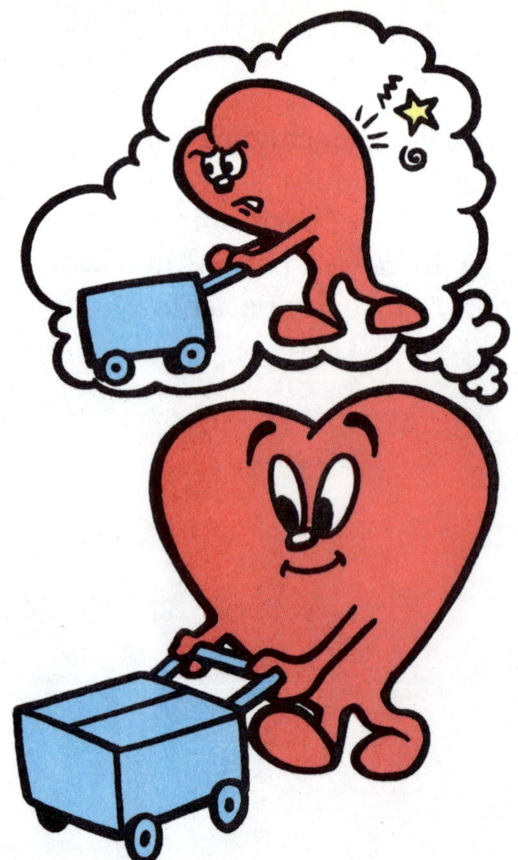

Procedure

1. Make sure you can handle the load. If not, call for assistance. Never try to lift too much by yourself.

2. Tell the patient what you are going to do.

3. Check your stance. Feet should be shoulder width apart, with knees bent, pointing in the direction of the move. Position your body in a straight line; do not twist or bend.

4. Hold the person or object you are lifting close to you, without stretching.

5. Keep your back straight, bend at the knees, and use your legs to lift.

6. When lifting with a team, count "1, 2, 3, LIFT," and make sure everyone lifts together smoothly. Stop if any team member is not ready or if the load shifts.

Safety is the primary concern in moving or positioning a patient.

Frequent positioning and good body alignment aid circulation, relieve pressure, and add to the patient's comfort. Some patients cannot or should not move themselves and need to be repositioned every hour or two. Always check the patient's care plan for frequency of positioning and any restrictions that may apply.

Two major problems for patients who are inactive are **contractures** (tightening of muscles) and **decubitus ulcers** (bedsores or pressure sores). Decubitus ulcers are painful and treatment is difficult. Prevention depends on frequent positioning, good nursing care, and careful observation. Watch for signs of pale or red skin color at pressure points, and report your observations if the color does not return to normal after pressure is relieved.

Positioning the Patient in Bed

Five common positions for bedridden patients are prone, supine, lateral, Sim's, and Fowler's.

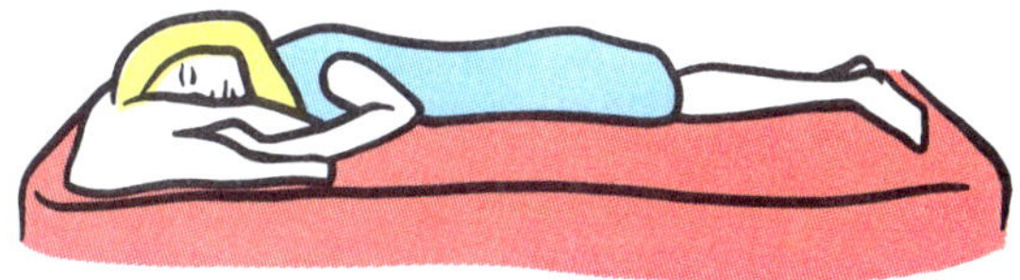

Prone
(lying on stomach)

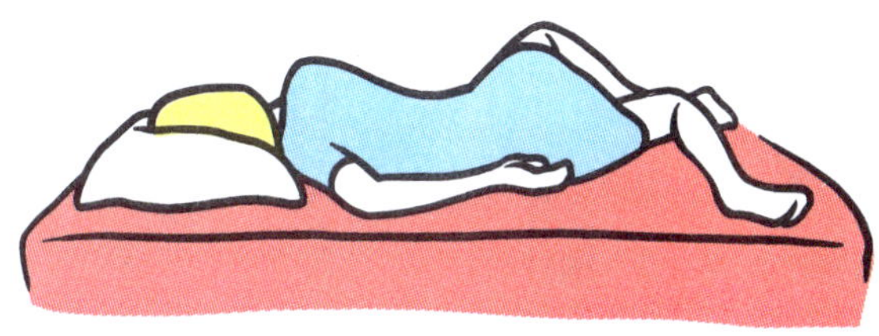

Sim's Position
(semi-prone, lying on the left side, with the right knee bent to the abdomen, the left knee bent slightly, left arm behind)

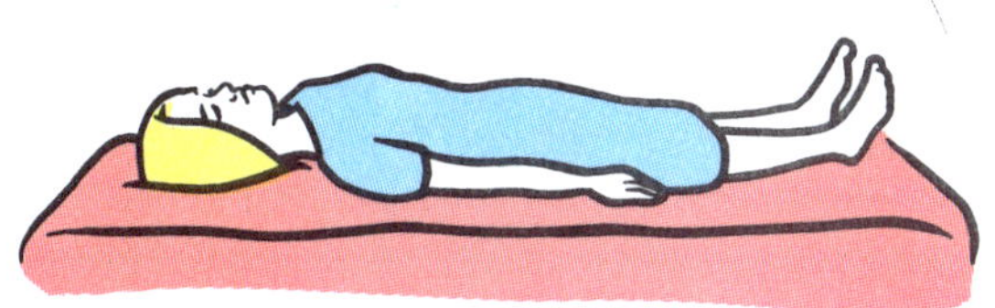

Supine
(lying on back)

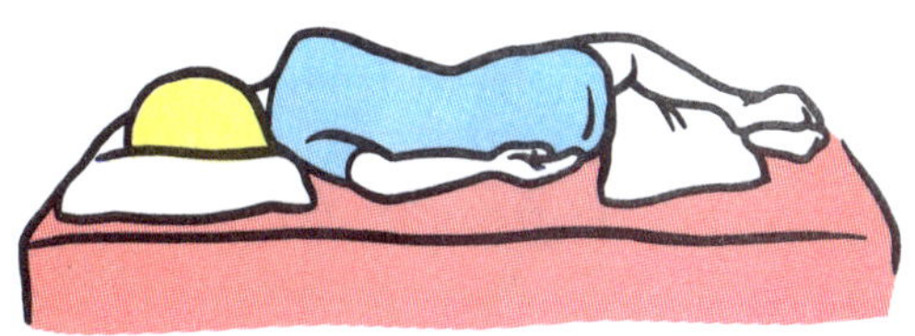

Lateral
(lying on side)

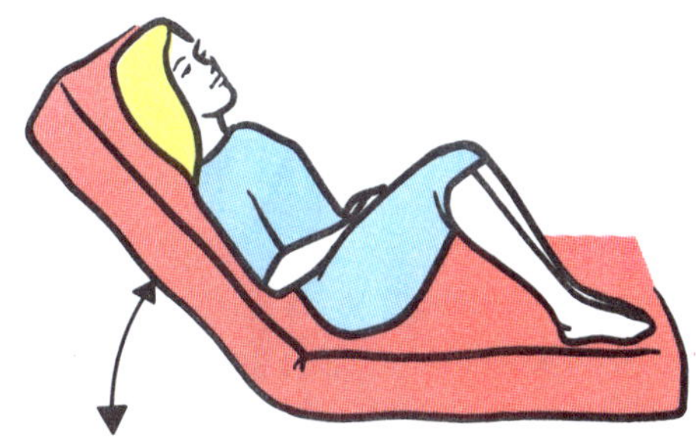

Fowler's Position
(sitting at 45⁰ angle with knees bent)
Semi-Fowler
(sitting at an angle less than 45⁰)

Incorrect Position

Positioning the Patient in a Chair

Proper alignment and positioning are important for patients when sitting. Make sure that the patient has good circulation at all times.

1. Be sure the patient's hips are pressing on the back of the chair.

2. Feet should rest comfortably on the floor or foot rest.

3. Position the back of the knees slightly away from the edge of the chair.

4. If necessary, ask permission from the nursing staff to place a pillow to support the patient's lower back.

5. Correct any slumping.
   - If the patient slumps sideways, place a pillow on that side for support and to straighten the spine.
   - If the patient slumps forward, align the spine by propping pillows on each side or in front.

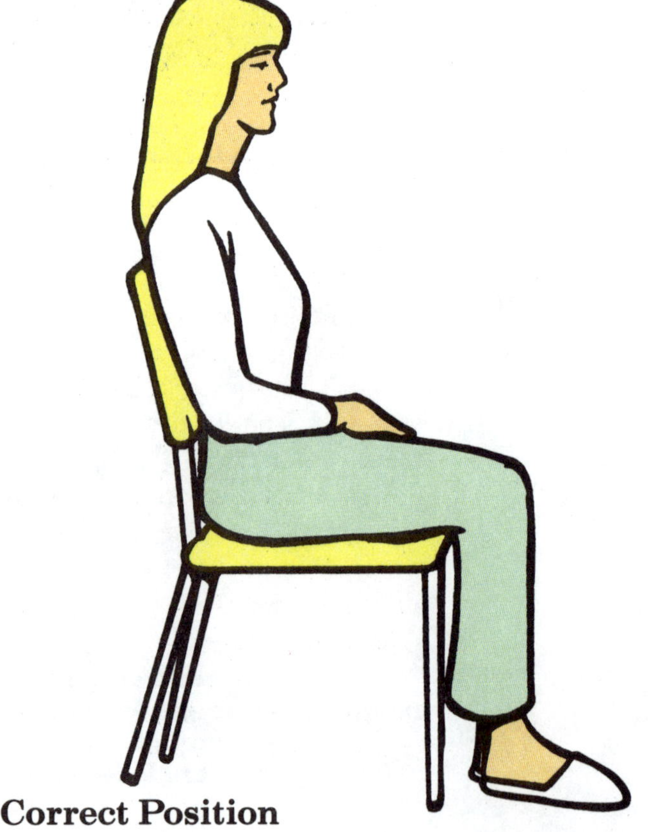

Correct Position

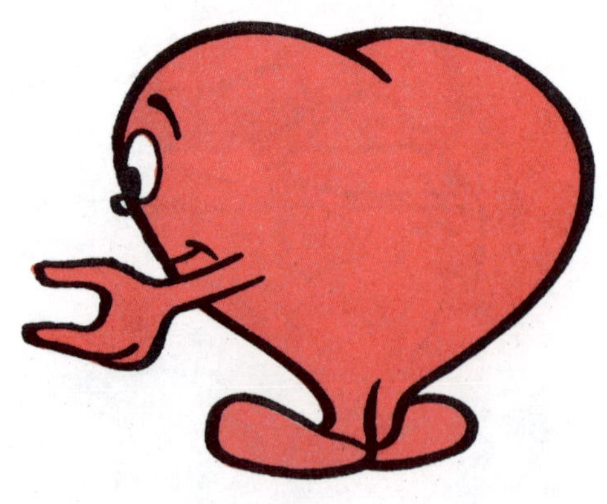

Part 3   # Moving

Check the care plan for any restrictions before moving a patient.

Prevent **friction** (rubbing one surface against another) when moving a patient. Roll or lift rather than sliding. Friction is painful and can damage the skin.

Moving Guidelines

1. Check identification to be sure you have the right patient.

2. Tell the patient what you are going to do.

3. Wash your hands before and after moving the patient.

4. Provide privacy.

5. Encourage the patient to help as much as possible.

6. Be sure all wheels are locked (bed, wheelchair).

7. The bed should be flat and at a level for good body mechanics.

8. Use good body mechanics, bending at the hips and knees with your back straight.

9. If you need assistance, be sure you have help before you begin.

10. After the move, position the patient properly, raise the side rails, and place the call signal within reach.

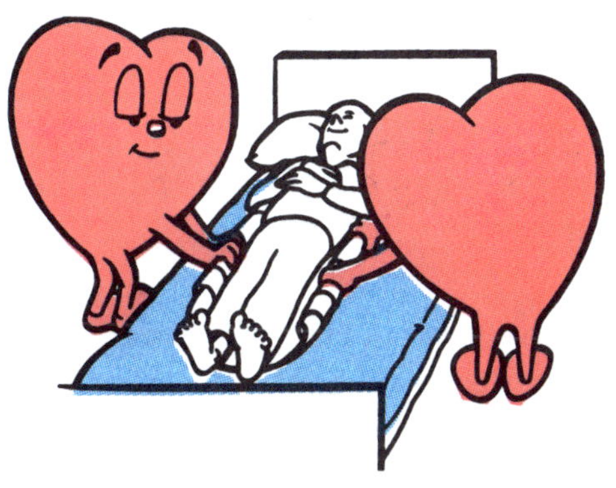

Moving the Patient Up in Bed

1. Put a pillow against the headboard to prevent injury.

2. Secure the side rail away from you and lower the one nearest you.

3. Put one arm under the patient's shoulders and the other arm under the thighs.

4. Have the patient put both feet flat on the bed and bend at the knees.

5. On the count of three, have the patient push with the feet while you lift toward the head of the bed.

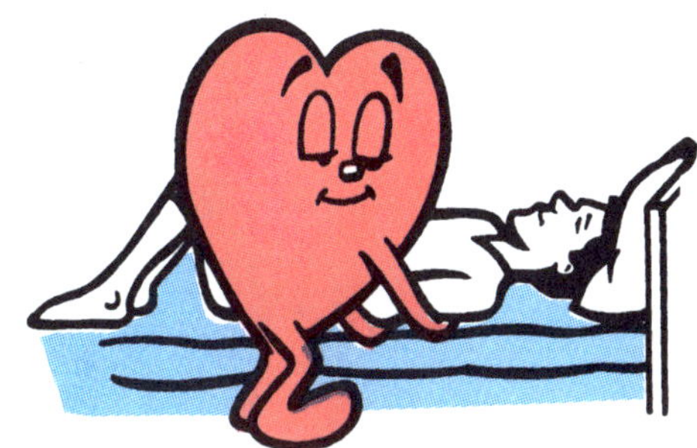

Moving with a Lift Sheet

A lift sheet is used to move patients who cannot help in any way or are very fragile. Never use a lift sheet without assistance.

1. You and your partner stand on opposite sides of the bed.

2. Lower the side rails.

3. Place a folded sheet under the patient from the shoulders to the knees.

4. Grip the sheet firmly at the patient's shoulders and hips.

5. On the count of three, lift the patient smoothly to the desired position.

Turning a Patient

Always turn a patient toward you if possible. Place one arm under the back and the other under the thigh as far as possible, and draw the patient toward you.

Turning a patient away from you may cause fear of falling because he or she cannot see you. Place one arm under the back and the other under the thigh as far as possible. Lift and draw the side away from you toward you. Gently turn the patient away from you.

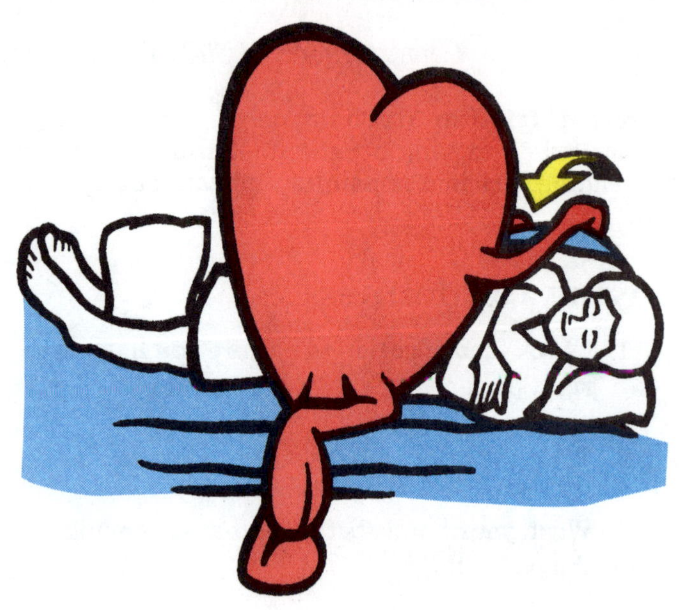

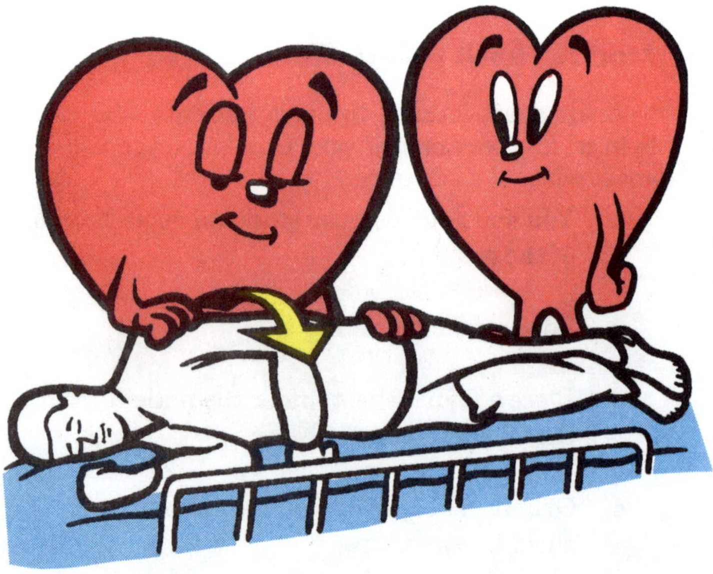

Log Rolling

A patient with spinal injuries must be moved without changing body alignment. The back, hips, and legs must be moved together, in straight alignment.

1. Make sure you have help.

2. Roll a lift sheet tightly to the patient's body.

3. Place a pillow between the patient's legs for support.

4. On the count of three, lift together, smoothly, to the desired side of the bed.

Part 4 — Transferring

Encourage the patient to help in the transfer as much as possible.

The NA **transfers** (moves from one place to another) patients many times a day:

- bed to wheelchair
- bed to commode (portable bedside toilet)
- bed to stretcher
- wheelchair to toilet
- wheelchair to tub or shower
- wheelchair to stretcher

The **pivot transfer** is used for patients who are **hemiplegic** (paralyzed on one side).

1. Identify the patient and explain what you are going to do.

2. Provide privacy.

3. Lock all wheels (bed, wheelchair).

4. Keep transfer sites close together, equalizing heights as much as possible.

5. Put the bed at its lowest position with the head raised to a sitting position.

6. Lower the side rail.

7. Help the patient to a sitting position with feet over the edge of the bed.

8. Stay with the patient and allow time to regain balance.

9. Assist with robe and slippers.

10. Stand in front of the patient, and put your arms under the patient's arms or use a transfer belt.

11. Put the paralyzed leg between your knees with your feet wide apart, and the patient's arms around your waist or shoulders (never around your neck).

12. Help the patient stand, supporting with your knees.

13. Slowly turn with the patient (without twisting), and gently lower the patient into the chair.

14. Position the patient properly.

To transfer the patient back into bed, reverse the procedure, making sure to raise the side rail and place the call signal within reach.

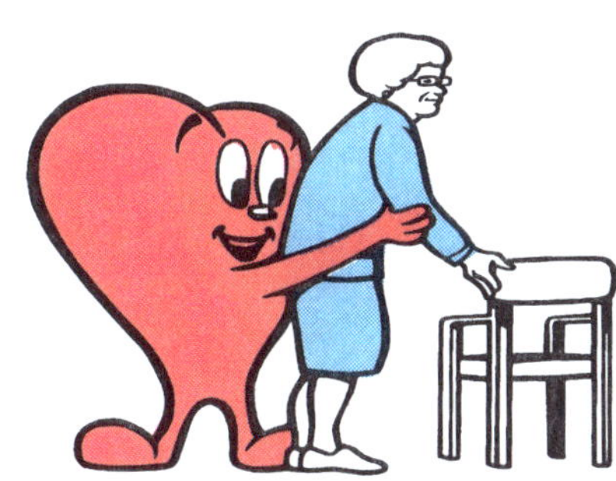

Active Transfer
(patient moves with minimal help)

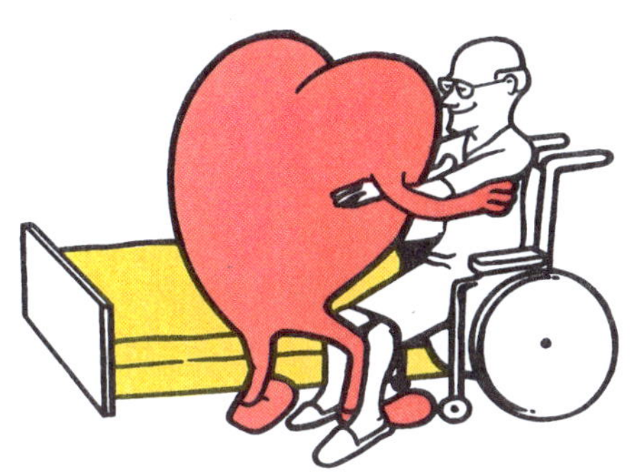

Assistive Transfer
(patient is able to help)

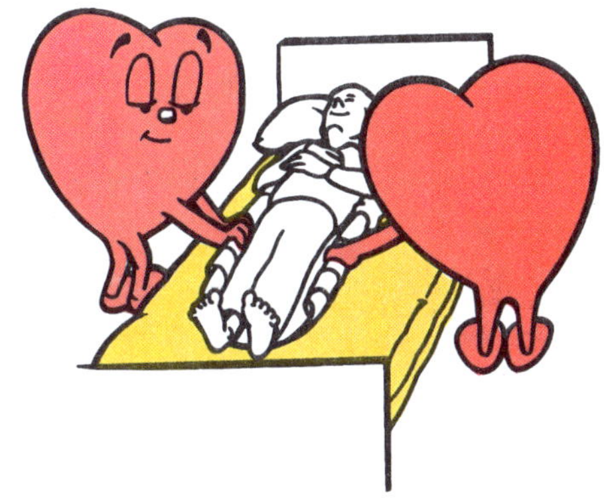

Passive Transfer
(patient is unable to help; at least two people are needed for the transfer)

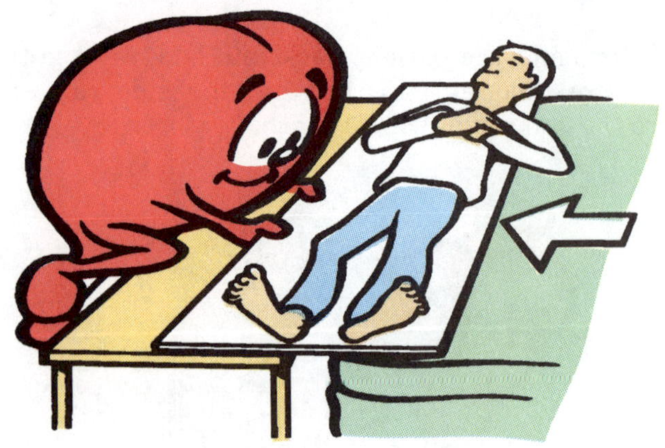

The transfer board keeps the back straight during transfer of a helpless patient. The transfer board is used when there is danger of spinal injury.

The drawsheet is used to transfer patients when there is no danger of back injury. For helpless patients, at least two NAs are required for the transfer.

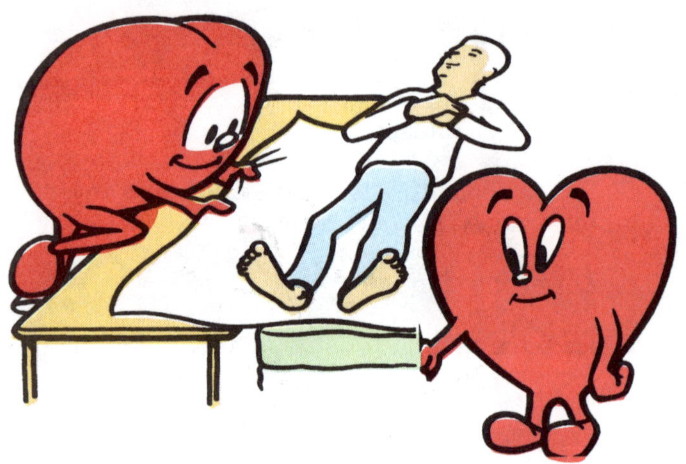

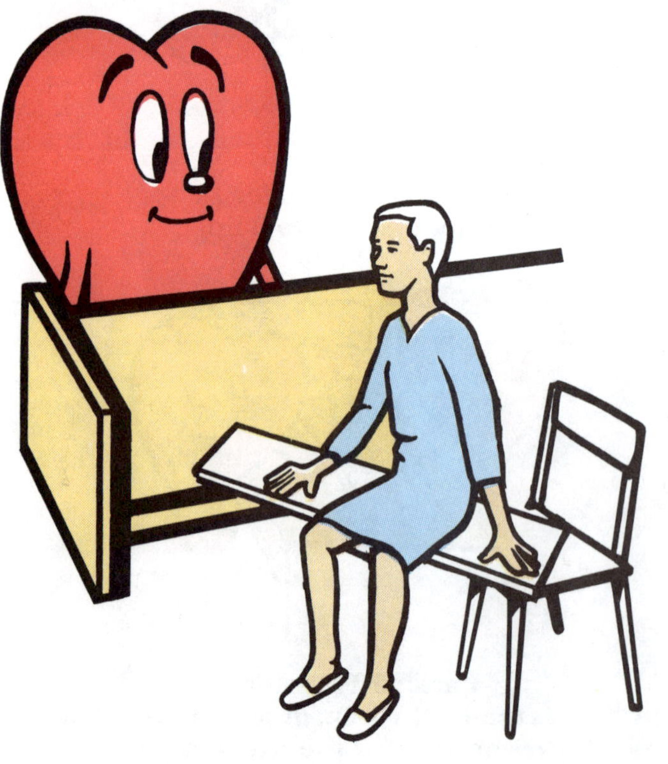

The slide board is a small board placed between the bed and the wheelchair. The patient sits on the board and is helped to slide across the board into the desired position. The slide board is used when there is no danger of spinal injury.

The transfer belt is placed around the patient's waist to provide a grip for the NA in transferring. It is used when transferring a semi-helpless or helpless patient. The belt is called a **gait belt** when used to assist in walking.

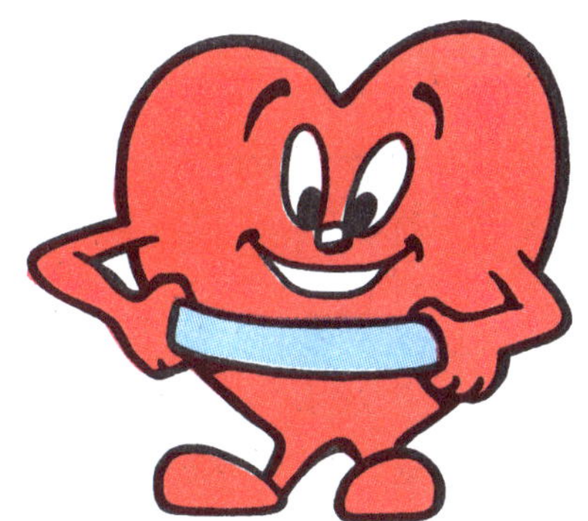

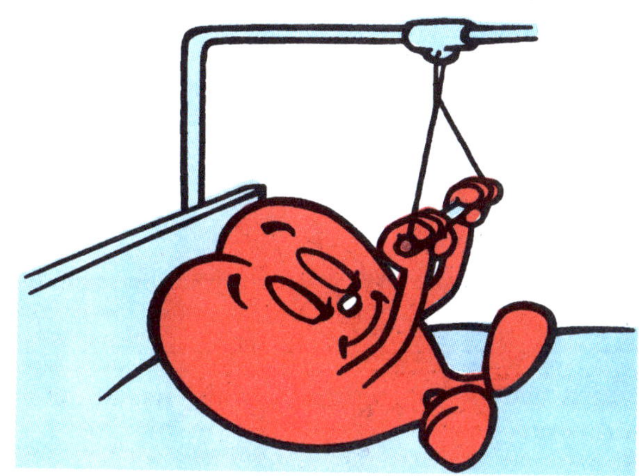

The trapeze bar is a swinging bar hanging over the bed from a metal frame. The patient grasps the bar with both hands and lifts the **torso** (top of the body) off the bed. The trapeze may be used for moving a patient up in bed, turning in bed, and to strengthen the arm muscles.

The hydraulic lift is used for patients who are too heavy to lift. **Always** have assistance when operating the hydraulic lift. Make sure you understand the operation. Ask your supervisor for help if you have any doubt. The lift is never used to transport a patient.

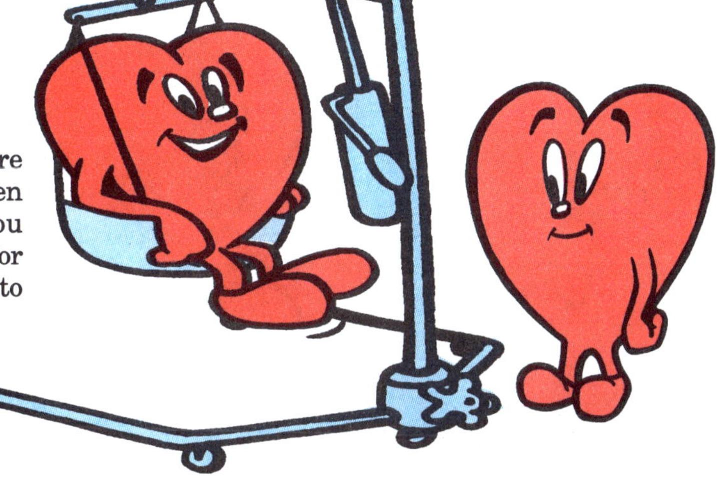

NA Review

1. Describe correct lifting procedures.

2. Identify three reasons why frequent repositioning is important.

   1.) To prevent bedsores.

3. How do you know when to reposition a patient?

4. What are good body mechanics, and why are they important for the NA?

5. Which transfer procedures require assistance, and why?

6. Explain when log rolling is necessary.

contracture	(kun-**track**-chur)	tightening of muscles
decubitus ulcer	(de-**kew**-bi-tus **ul**-ser)	bedsore
hemiplegic	(hem-i-**plee**-jick)	paralyzed on one side
supine	(suh-**pine**)	lying on back
transfer	(**trans**-fur)	to move from one place to another

Additional Terms to Remember

NA Notes

Use proper lifting techniques to prevent injuries.

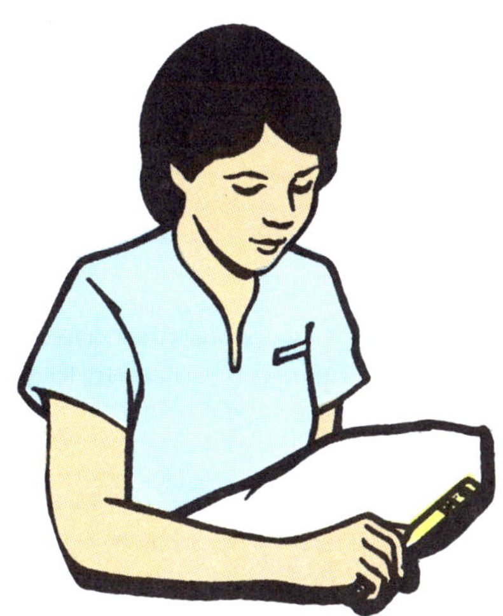

Taking Vital Signs

Accurate measurements help determine a patient's condition!

Objectives:

- ☐ Name the four vital signs
- ☐ Identify three locations for taking temperature
- ☐ Identify the pulse points
- ☐ Demonstrate how to take and record blood pressure
- ☐ Discuss proper procedures for counting respirations

<table><tr><td>Part 1</td><td>

Temperature
</td></tr></table>

Body heat provides important health information.

Temperature, pulse, respiration, and blood pressure (TPR/BP) are called **vital signs** (V.S.). The NA needs to know how to measure V.S. Accurate measurements provide important health information for proper care.

Temperature (T) refers to body heat and is measured with a digital or glass thermometer.

There are two parts of the thermometer:

- **bulb** (the part that contacts the patient's body)
- **stem** (the part showing the display)

Three body areas for measuring temperature and the average ranges in **Fahrenheit** (F) and **Celsius** (C):

- **oral** (mouth) 95^0 - 98^0F   (35^0 - 36.6^0C)
- **axillary** (armpit) 94^0 - 97^0F   (34.4^0 - 36^0 C)
- **rectal** (anus) 96^0 - 99^0F   (35.5^0 - 37.2^0C)

Glass Thermometers

Glass thermometers are hollow glass tubes filled with **mercury** (a liquid metal). The stem is **calibrated** (marked) in degrees and fractions of degrees. Care must be taken not to drop glass thermometers because they break easily.

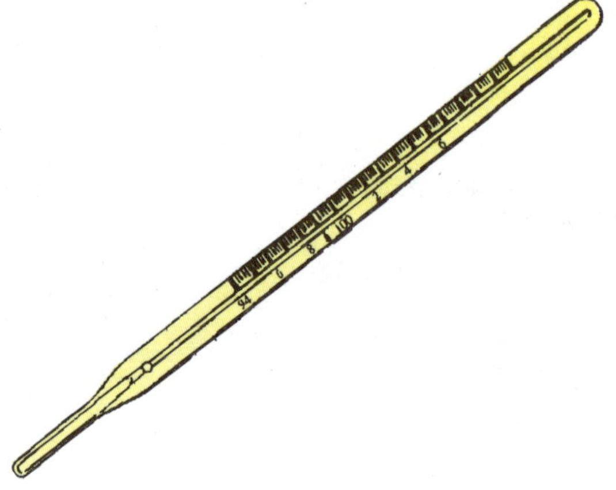

Oral Glass Thermometer

Never clean a glass thermometer with hot water. The mercury will expand and the thermometer may break.

Soak the thermometer in disinfectant. Rinse it in cool water before placing in the patient's mouth.

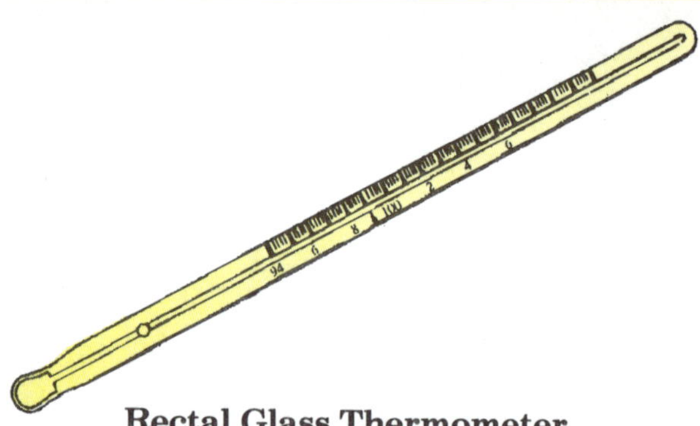

Rectal Glass Thermometer

Digital Thermometers

Digital thermometers show the temperature in a digital display. They do not require "shaking down" like glass thermometers.

Cover the mouth piece with a clear plastic sheath. Dispose of the sheath after each use.

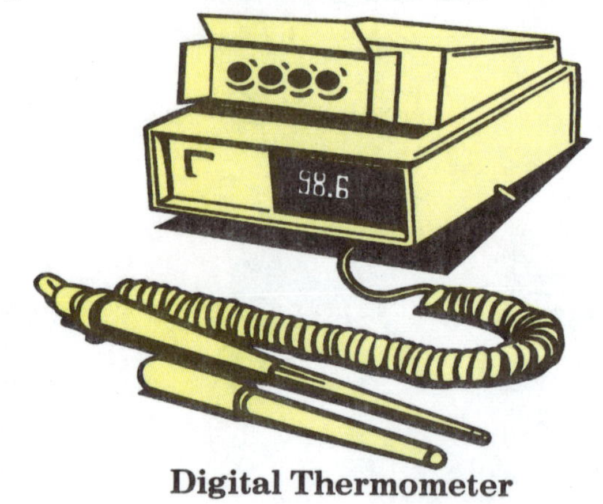

Digital Thermometer

Oral Temperatures

Digital/Oral

Oral temperatures are taken when a patient has no difficulty holding a thermometer in the mouth.

Never take an oral temperature if a person:

- cannot breathe with the mouth closed.
- is unconscious.
- is six years or younger.
- has seizures.
- is on oxygen.

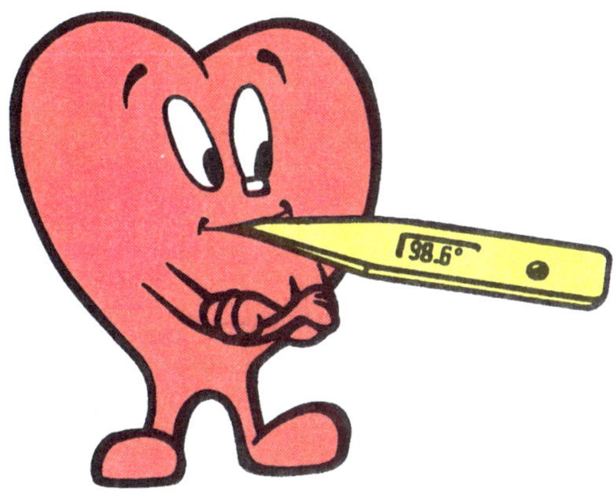

Procedure

1. Wash your hands.

2. Hold the thermometer by the stem (never touch the bulb).

3. Place a disposable sleeve over the stem.

4. Tell the patient what you are going to do.

5. Gently insert the bulb end under the patient's tongue.

6. Ask the patient to keep the lips closed.

7. Leave the thermometer in place for 20 seconds or until the beep.

Never leave a patient unattended with a thermometer in place.

8. Remove and read the display.

9. Evaluate the reading. If it seems low, retake the temperature.

10. Discard the disposable sleeve.

11. Record the temperature in the patient's chart.

12. Report major changes from previous readings.

13. Wash your hands.

Glass/Oral

An oral thermometers has a slender bulb. Never use a glass thermometer when someone is confused and might bite down on it.

Procedure

Follow the same procedure as a digital thermometer with these exceptions:

- Inspect the thermometer for chips and cracks.

- Keep a firm grip and shake the mercury down the stem into the bulb.

- Leave the thermometer in place for three minutes.

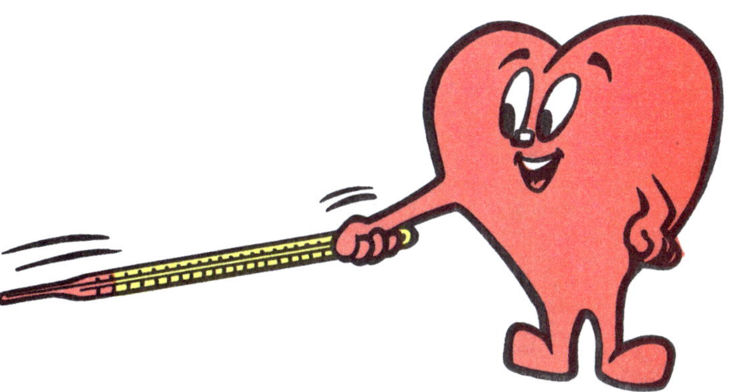

Rectal Temperatures

Digital/Rectal

Procedure

Use the same procedure as an oral temperature with the following exceptions:

- Lubricate the bulb with petroleum jelly.

- Insert the bulb one inch into the rectum, and hold in place for 10 seconds or until the beep.

- Remove and wipe with a tissue.

- Read the temperature and record.

Glass/Rectal

Be sure you have a *rectal* thermometer when using glass thermometers for rectal temperatures. Rectal thermometers have a rounder bulb to prevent injury during insertion. The bulb is often colored red for easy identification.

Procedure

Use the same procedure as a digital thermometer, except leave in place for three minutes.

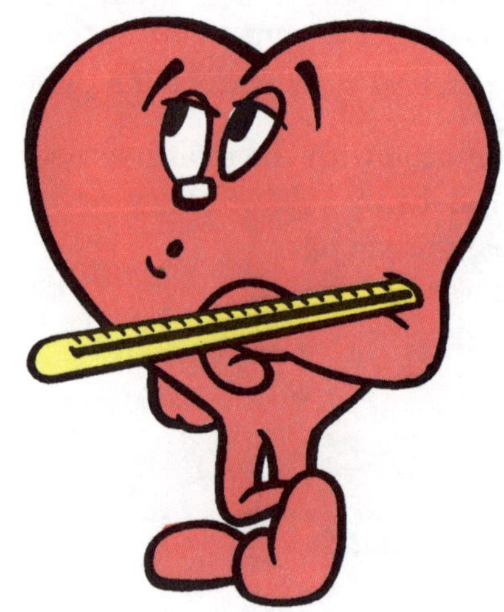

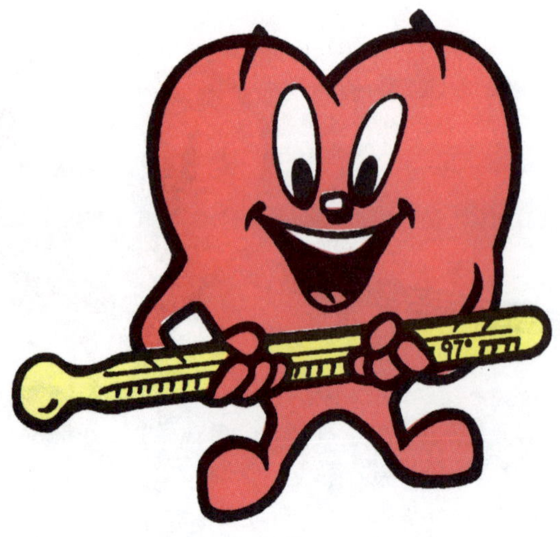

Axillary Temperatures

Digital/Axillary

Procedure

Follow the same procedure as an oral temperature with these exceptions:

- Place the thermometer in the center of the **axilla** (armpit).

- Put the patient's arm across his or her chest to hold the thermometer in place.

- Wait for the beep.

Glass/Axillary

Be sure to use an *oral* thermometer for axillary temperatures.

Procedure

Follow the same procedures as for a digital axillary temperature, except hold in place for 10 minutes.

Part 2   # Pulse

*As the heart beats, it pumps blood into the arteries,
causing them to expand and contract.*

The heart's contractions (pulse) are measured to determine how fast the heart is beating. The average range for adults is 56 - 80 **beats per minute** (bpm).

When measuring the pulse, observe three things:

- **rate** (number of beats per minute)
- **rhythm** (how regular and even the beats are)
- **strength** (weak or pounding)

Compare your observations with previously recorded rates and report any differences.

The pulse can be felt easily at the points of the body where the arteries are closest to the skin. The three most common points are radial, carotid, and apical.

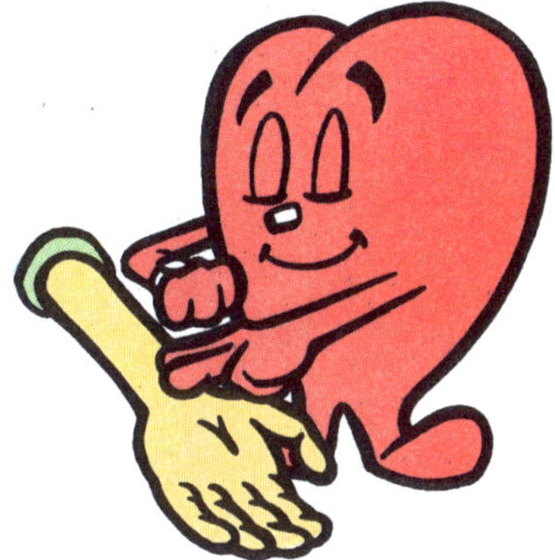

Radial (thumb side)

The wrist is where the **radial pulse** (from the radial artery) is felt. If the pulse is very weak, take a reading from the other arm for comparison.

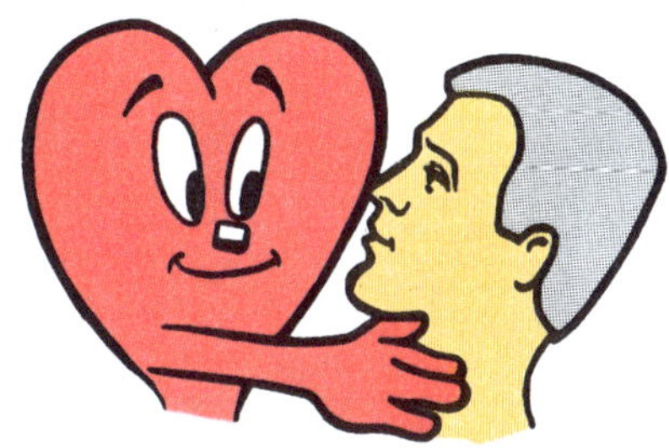

Carotid

The **carotid artery** is in the neck, next to the Adam's apple, and can be felt when the pulse is too weak to feel at the wrist.

Apical

An **apical** pulse is a measurement of the heartbeats at the apex of the heart, under the left breast. A stethoscope is needed to hear the apical pulse.

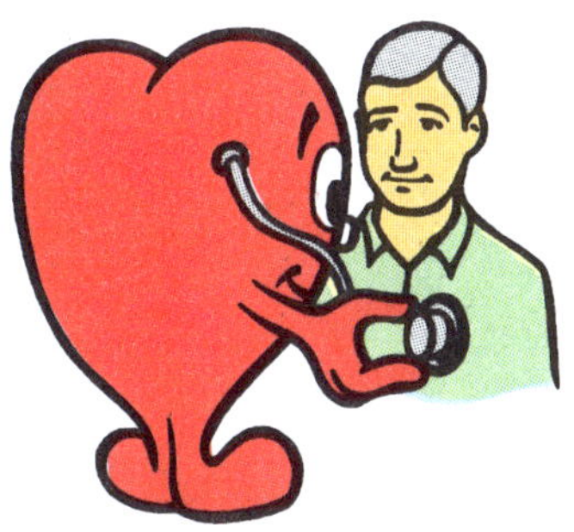

Other Pulse Sites

- temporal (temples)
- brachial (inside elbow)
- femoral (groin)
- popliteal (knee)
- pedal (top front shin)

Procedure

1. Measure the pulse when the patient is *at rest*. (Exercise, fever, emotions, or pain can increase the pulse rate.)

2. Locate the pulse.

3. Using a watch with a second hand, count the beats for 30 seconds and multiply by two for the bpm pulse rate.

4. If the beat is irregular, count the beats for a full minute.

5. Record the pulse count.

6. Report major changes from previous readings.

<table><tr><td>Part 3</td><td><h1>Respiration</h1></td></tr></table>

Changes in breathing may be warning signs of respiratory problems.

Each **respiration** (breath) has two parts:

- **inspiration** (breathing in)
- **expiration** (breathing out)

To count respirations, watch or feel the patient's chest rise and fall.

Try to observe respirations without the patient's awareness to prevent any anxiety that might cause a change in the normal rate.

If possible, observe respirations while carrying on a conversation.

Some causes of increased respiration:

- fever
- exercise
- stress
- disease
- medications

Some causes of decreased respiration:

- medications
- disease

Adults average **16 - 20 respirations per minute.** Pay special attention to respirations that are:

- very fast or very slow
- noisy (describe the sound)
- shallow (very little chest movement)
- rapid
- labored (wheezing or with **great effort**)
- irregular

Notify your supervisor of any irregularities in breathing.

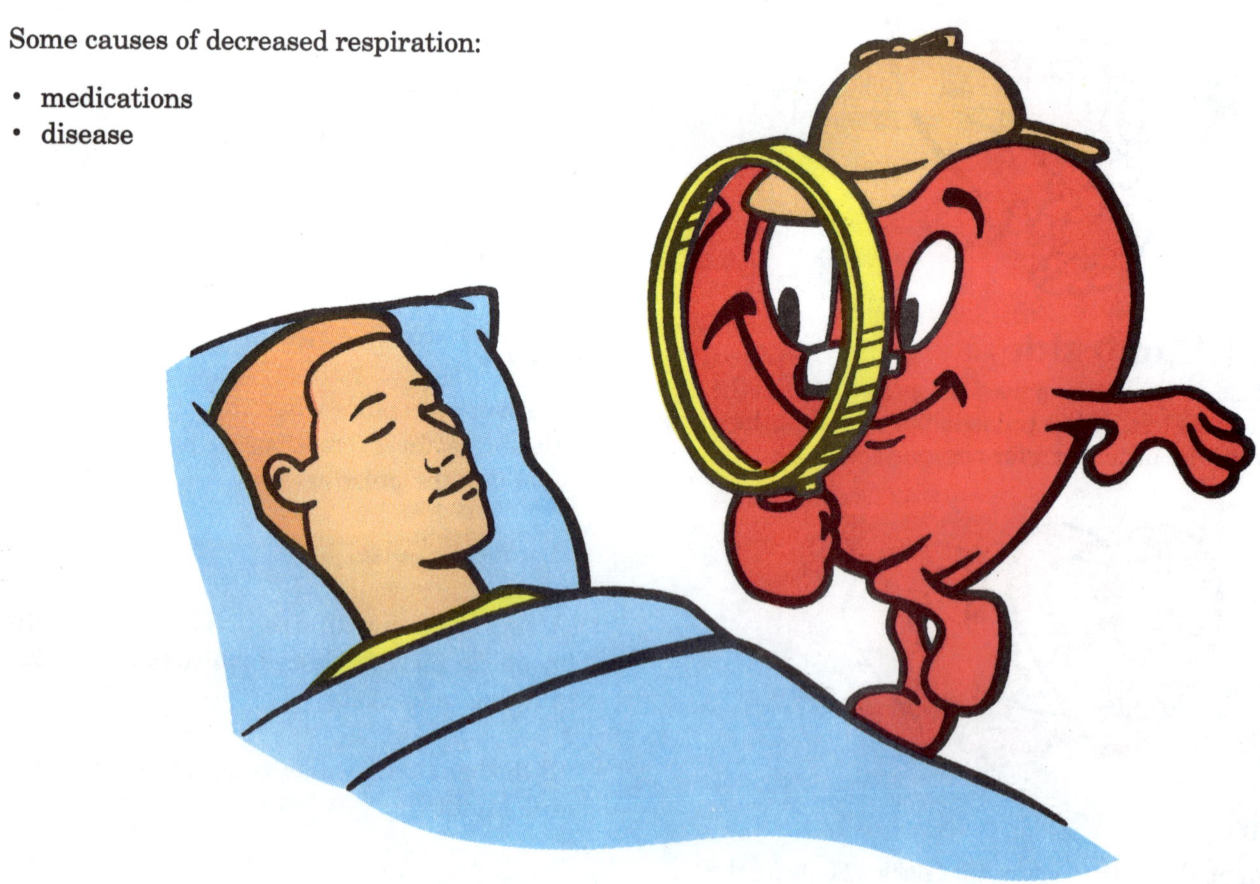

Part 4 — Blood Pressure

*The heart pumps blood through the circulatory system,
creating pressure against the arterial walls.*

Blood pressure (BP) readings provide valuable information for the care and treatment of the patient.

A patient's blood pressure should be taken each time with the patient in the same position, preferably sitting. The BP is taken with a sphygmomanometer (blood pressure cuff) and a stethoscope.

The BP consists of two measurements:
- **systolic pressure** (when the heart contracts)
- **diastolic pressure** (when the heart relaxes)

The systolic pressure is the highest and is heard first. The normal range is 100 - 140 measured in **millimeters** (mm) of mercury.

The diastolic is the pressure when the heart is relaxed. The normal range is 60 - 90 mm.

When recording blood pressure, the systolic is written above the diastolic. An example of a normal BP would be written 120/70.

Hypertension is high blood pressure:

- systolic above 150 mm
- diastolic above 90 mm

Elderly people tend to have higher BP readings due to **arteriosclerosis** (loss of elasticity in the arteries) or **cerebral vascular accident** (CVA or stroke).

BP may increase due to:

- kidney disease
- exercise
- medications
- stress
- obesity
- pain

Hypotension is low blood pressure. BP decreases with:
- hemorrhage
- medications
- rest
- heart disease
- **shock** (sudden disturbance of body functions affecting blood circulation)

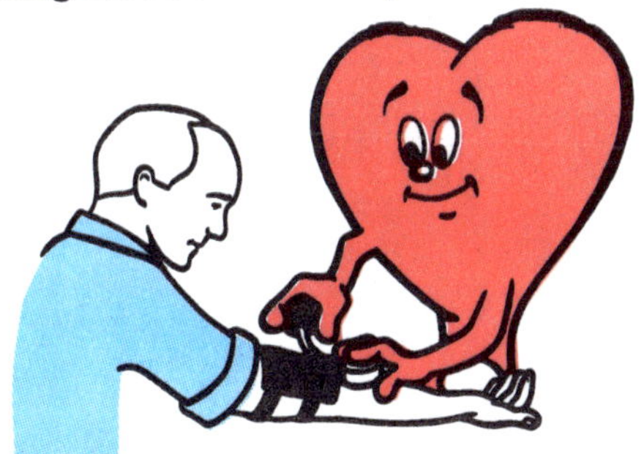

Procedure

1. Wash your hands.

2. Explain what you are going to do.

3. Wrap the BP cuff snugly around the patient's bare arm, two inches above the elbow.

4. Locate the brachial pulse (inside elbow).

5. Place the stethoscope diaphragm over the pulse.

6. Close the valve and inflate the cuff until you no longer feel the pulse. Note the number.

7. Inflate the cuff to 30 mm above this number.

8. Open the valve and let air escape slowly until the pulse is heard.

9. Note the systolic pressure (the number corresponding to the first sound you hear).

10. Let the air out further and listen for the last sound you can hear.

11. Note the diastolic pressure.

12. Record systolic/diastolic readings.

13. Wait 30 seconds and repeat the procedure to check your readings. If the BP is unusually low, take a reading from the other arm for comparison.

14. Deflate and remove the cuff.

15. Cleanse the stethoscope with an alcohol swab.

16. Wash your hands.

17. Record the blood pressure in the patient's record.

18. Report major changes from previous readings.

NA Review

1. Describe the difference between oral and rectal thermometers, and when you should use each type.

   ____

   ____

   ____

   ____

2. Why is it important to inspect glass thermometers before using them?

   ____

   ____

   ____

   ____

3. Identify three common areas for measuring the pulse.

   ____

   ____

   ____

4. Name three observations to make while measuring pulse.

   1.) Strength of the beat

   ____

   ____

5. What could cause an increase in respiration?

   ____

   ____

   ____

6. What could cause a patient's BP to be higher than normal, and what would you do about it?

   ____

   ____

   ____

   ____

Vocabulary

apical	(**ap**-i-kul)	pulse point to the left of the breast bone
arteriosclerosis	(ahr-teer-ee-o-**skle**-**ro**-sis)	hardening of the arteries
axillary	(**ack**-si-ler-ee)	in the armpit
brachial	(**bra**-ke-ul)	pulse point at the inside elbow
carotid	(ka-**rot**-id)	pulse point on each side of the neck
diastolic	(dy-a-**stol**-ick)	blood pressure when heart relaxes
expiration	(eck-spi-**ray**-shun)	breathing out
femoral	(**fem**-or-ul)	pulse point in groin (where the abdomen joins the thigh)
hemorrhage	(**hem**-uh-rij)	bleeding
hypertension	(hy-pur-**ten**-shun)	blood pressure higher than normal
hypotension	(hy-po-**ten**-shun)	blood pressure lower than normal
inspiration	(in-spi-**ray**-shun)	breathing in
oral	(**or**-ul)	pertaining to the mouth
pedal	(**ped**-ul)	pulse point at top front of shin
popliteal	(pop-**lit**-e-ul)	pulse point at back of knee
radial	(**ray**-dee-ul)	pulse point in the wrist
rectal	(**reck**-tul)	pertaining to the anus
respiration	(res-per-**ay**-shun)	breathing
systolic	(sis-**tol**-ick)	pressure created when heart contracts
sphygmomanometer	(sfig-mo-ma-**nom**-e-tur)	blood pressure cuff

Additional Terms to Remember

NA Notes

Always stay with the patient when using a thermometer.

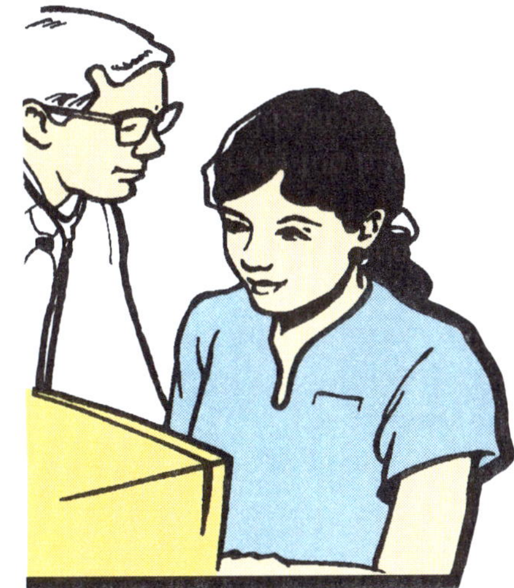

Basic Patient Care

Good skills earn the respect of patients and co-workers!

Objectives:

- ☐ Demonstrate accurate observing, reporting, charting
- ☐ Demonstrate good oral hygiene techniques
- ☐ Explain procedures for hair and nail care
- ☐ Identify three methods of bathing
- ☐ Demonstrate proper bedmaking
- ☐ Demonstrate weighing and measuring techniques

Part 1 Observing, Reporting, and Charting

*The health-care team depends on the NA's accurate
and timely reports to manage each patient's care.*

Three important responsibilities of the NA are observing, reporting, and charting.

Observing

Learn to observe the patient
throughout your daily contacts.

Being a skilled observer helps prevent serious problems and earns the respect of the nursing staff. Being alert to the patient and the environment reduces safety hazards and health problems. Careful observation increases your awareness of the patient's physical, emotional, and social needs.

Learn to recognize signs and symptoms of common diseases and conditions. One of the major keys to helping a patient is detecting a problem in its early stages.

Watch. Look. Listen. Trust your instincts. If something seems to be wrong, report it.

Physical Changes

- decreased or increased functioning (elimination, pulse, breathing, etc.)
- unconscious, weak, dizzy, shaking, trembling
- dopey, drowsy, lethargic
- cold, pale, clammy
- hot, sweating, burning, feverish
- nausea, vomiting
- diarrhea, constipation
- excessive thirst
- odor
- ringing in ears
- blurred vision
- spasms
- pain, difficulty
- swelling, edema
- rash, hives, blisters
- choking, coughing, wheezing, sneezing

Emotional Changes

- mood swings, loss of control
- depressed, hopeless, crying, tearful
- angry, difficult, irrational
- disoriented, confused
- anxious, frightened, pacing

Reporting

Thorough and accurate reports are made to the nursing staff as often as the patient's condition requires. End-of-shift reports to the on-coming staff provide the information necessary for continued good care.

Reports should include:

- the patient's name.
- room and bed number.
- detailed description of the observation.

Objective reporting means to report precisely what you see, smell, feel, or hear. If a patient complains of symptoms that you cannot observe, such as dizziness or pain, report exactly what the patient tells you.

Correct:	Mrs. Smith said her left ear aches, as reported to the **charge nurse** (CN).
Correct:	Mrs. Jones's right arm is red, swollen, and warm to the touch.

Subjective reporting is used to report what you cannot sense. The NA should avoid using subjective reporting. However, if you think something is wrong medically or emotionally, report it to the CN and chart the report. Report any patient complaints immediately.

Incorrect:	Mrs. Smith has an ear infection.
Correct:	Mrs. Smith says her ear aches, and she seems very uncomfortable, as reported to the CN.

Charting

To chart a patient's record:

- Write notes on paper first, then check for accuracy and spelling.

- Write clearly and neatly in ink.

- Correct errors by drawing a single line through the error and signing it. Never erase or "white-out" a record.

- Always write the date and time of the notation.

- Chart only procedures that you have done, after they are done.

- Chart reports of observations.

- Always sign the entry.

- Keep all information confidential.

The chart is the written health record of the patient. It is a legal document. Accuracy is very important!

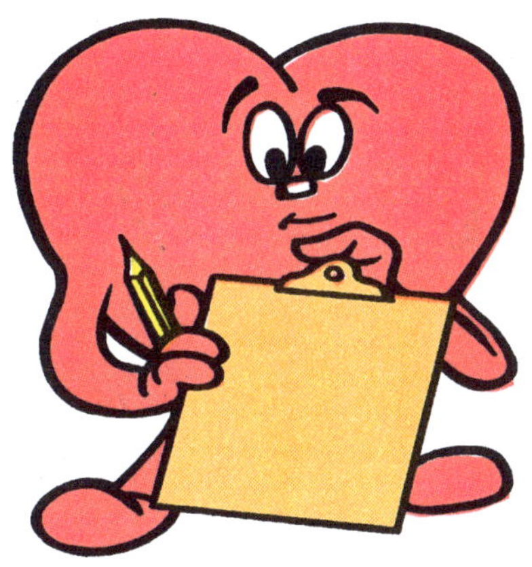

Part 2   Promoting Independence

Help patients maintain their independence by
focusing on their abilities, not disabilities.

One of the biggest challenges in long-term care is helping patients to be independent. Encouraging patients to do something for themselves may take more effort than doing it for them.

Older people have the same basic needs they had when they were younger. They want to feel useful and to keep as much control of their lives as they can. The more you do for the patients that they could do themselves, the more you take away control and contribute to their decline.

Activities of daily living (ADL) such as walking, dressing, eating, and bathing may become increasingly difficult with age. Familiarize yourself with self-care devices that allow the patient to be independent, such as special eating utensils and aids for dressing and grooming.

The goal of long-term care is to **rehabilitate** (restore what has been lost). The health-care team develops individual care plans based on what is possible for each patient. The plan encourages independence and promotes the highest level of physical, mental, and emotional wellness. Patients have the right to participate in decisions about their care, and the team encourages them to make personal choices.

Part 3 — Bed Making

A properly made bed adds to the patient's comfort and well-being.

Part of the NA's daily routine is bed making. A properly made bed is free of wrinkles that cause discomfort and painful bedsores.

Making an Unoccupied Bed

1. Wash your hands before and after handling linens.

2. Gather the linens:
   - mattress pad
   - plastic drawsheet
   - top sheet
   - bedspread
   - bottom sheet
   - cotton drawsheet
   - blanket
   - pillowcase

3. Raise the bed to a level for good body mechanics.

4. Place the mattress pad on the bed.

5. Unfold and lay the bottom sheet so it hangs evenly on both sides.

6. Tuck the top of the sheet under the mattress.

7. Make a **mitered** corner:
   - Raise the side of the sheet.
   - Lay it on top of the mattress.
   - Form a triangle.
   - Tuck the hanging portion under the mattress.
   - Bring the triangle down.
   - Tuck under the mattress.

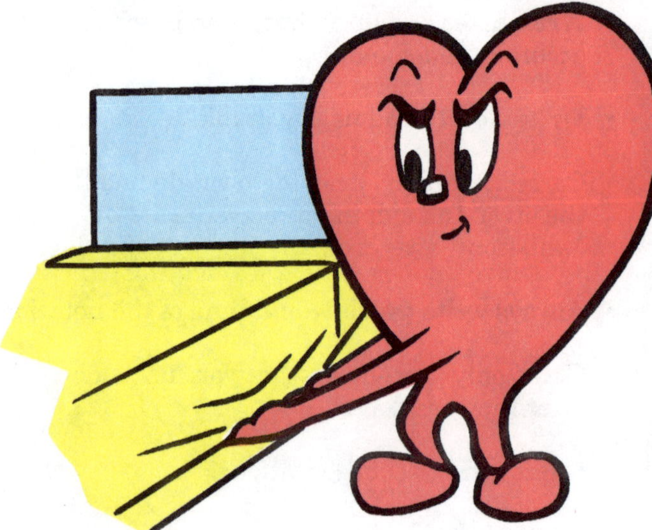

8. If a plastic drawsheet is used, place it on the bed.

9. Place the cotton drawsheet over the plastic drawsheet. Be sure to cover the plastic completely.

10. Tuck both drawsheets under the mattress.

11. Place the top sheet on the bed and miter the corners at the foot. Do not tuck the bottom under the mattress.

12. Place the blanket, then the bedspread, on the bed.

13. Tuck in the top sheet, blanket, and bedspread together, making mitered corners.

14. Move to the opposite side and repeat, pulling linens tightly to remove wrinkles.

15. Open the pillowcase. Guide the pillow in with seam end first. Do not hold the pillow under your chin!

16. Fold extra material under the pillow.

17. Place the pillow on the bed.

18. Place the call light within easy reach.

Making an Occupied Bed

The method for making an occupied bed is the same as making an unoccupied bed with these exceptions:

1. Obtain help, if needed.

2. Tell the patient what you are going to do.

3. Provide privacy.

4. Remove the bed linens, leaving the top sheet to cover the patient.

5. Turn the patient to the opposite side, away from you. **Be sure the side rail is up and locked!**

6. Roll the linens toward the patient and tuck the linens under his or her back.

7. Unfold and place clean linens with the center crease in the center of the bed.

8. Tuck in with mitered corners.

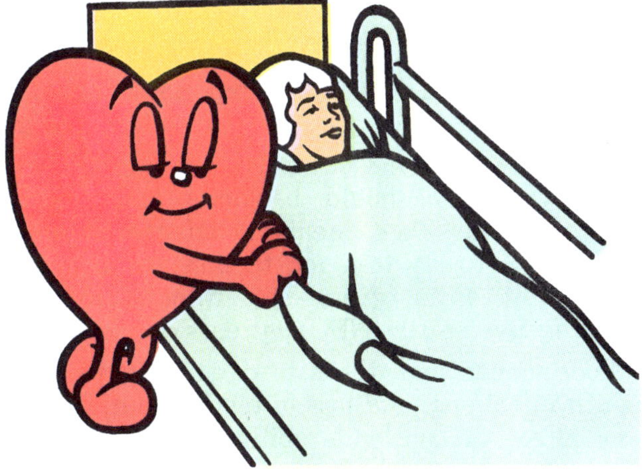

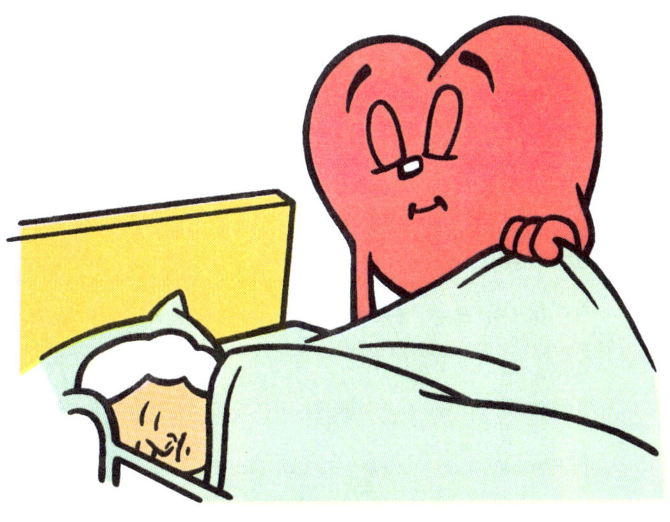

9. Raise the side rail where you have been working.

10. Move to the opposite side.

11. Lower the bed rail and roll the patient away from you onto the clean linens.

12. Remove soiled linens and repeat the process, pulling linens tight.

13. Place the clean top sheet over the patient and pull the soiled sheet from below, keeping the patient covered.

14. Replace the blankets and bedspread.

15. Change the pillowcase.

16. Position the patient comfortably and raise both side rails.

17. Place the call light within easy reach.

Part 4 — **Personal Hygiene**

Cleanliness promotes good health, and looking good boosts morale.

Personal hygiene (cleanliness) includes good care of the mouth, hair, nails, and skin.

Mouth Care

Brushing teeth is the most important part of **oral** (mouth) hygiene, but good care extends to the gums and tongue.

Oral hygiene should be done each morning, evening, and after meals. Patients should be encouraged to do this for themselves if possible. Mouth care is given to unconscious and **nothing-by-mouth** (NPO) patients every two hours.

Poor mouth care leads to cavities, gum disease, mouth infections, and loss of teeth. Mouth problems may affect the patient's ability and desire to eat, resulting in poor nutrition or insufficient fluid intake. Report any redness, sores, or bleeding to your supervisor.

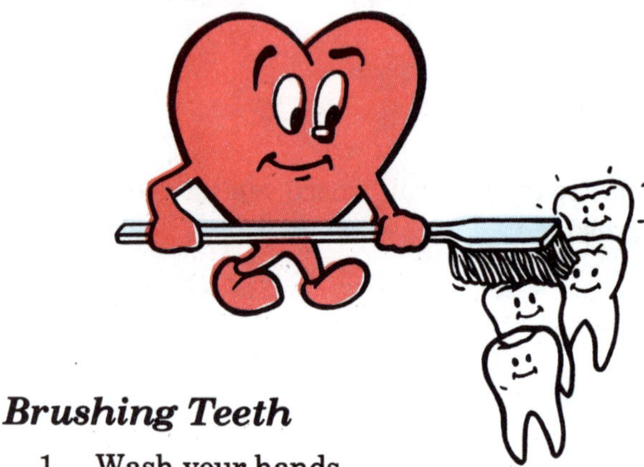

Brushing Teeth

1. Wash your hands.

2. Assemble equipment:
   - cup
   - mouthwash
   - emesis basin
   - water
   - soft toothbrush
   - towel
   - toothpaste

3. Explain what you are going to do.

4. Provide privacy.

5. Put on gloves.

6. Hold the toothbrush at a 45-degree angle to the gums.

7. Massage the gums by brushing in a circular motion where teeth and gums meet.

8. Brush the tongue.

9. Rinse well, and dry the patient's mouth.

10. Make sure the patient is comfortable.

11. Replace side rails.

12. Remove and dispose of gloves.

13. Report any problems to your supervisor (swollen gums, irritations, etc.).

For the unconscious patient, follow the same procedure with a few additional steps. Always explain what you are going to do. The patient may be able to hear you even though he or she is unable to respond.

- Add swabs and a water soluble lubricant to your equipment.

- Place a towel under the patient's face and put a basin by the mouth.

- Use swabs to clean the mouth, and a toothbrush for the teeth and tongue.

- Dry the lips and apply lubricant.

- Be careful to avoid **aspiration** (breathing into the lungs) of the lubricant.

Flossing

Flossing removes **plaque** (bacteria) that the toothbrush misses. Teeth should be flossed once a day before brushing. Follow the procedures for brushing through step 5. Assist only as needed.

- Tear off a piece of floss 12 - 15 inches long.

- Wrap the ends around the first or second finger of each hand, with the fingers not more than one-half inch apart.

- Slide the floss gently between the teeth, and move it up and down carefully three or four times against each tooth (without cutting the gums).

- Move to a fresh section of floss, and continue the process until all of the teeth have been flossed.

- Discard used floss.

- Proceed with brushing step 6.

Denture Care

Some patients wear full **dentures** (false teeth), or **partials** (removable artificial teeth that attach to permanent teeth). As a person ages, mouth tissues change, and dentures may need to be refitted. If a patient complains of discomfort or develops mouth sores, notify your supervisor.

Remove dentures or partials from the mouth at least eight hours a day, and store them in liquid to prevent warping. Rinse after meals and snacks, and clean thoroughly once a day. Assist the patient as needed.

1. Wash your hands.
2. Assemble equipment:
   * basin
   * soft denture brush
   * standard soft toothbrush
   * drinking glass
3. Tell the patient what you are going to do and provide privacy.
4. Wear gloves.
5. Remove the dentures and soak them in cleaner.
6. With dentures removed, clean the patient's mouth. Use a standard soft toothbrush to gently clean the tongue, and rinse the mouth thoroughly.
7. Fill the basin with warm (not hot) water, and hold the dentures over the water to avoid breaking if dropped.
8. Use a soft denture brush to clean the dentures. Never use a sharp tool for cleaning.
9. Store in liquid or insert in the patient's mouth.
10. Follow steps 8 - 13 for brushing.

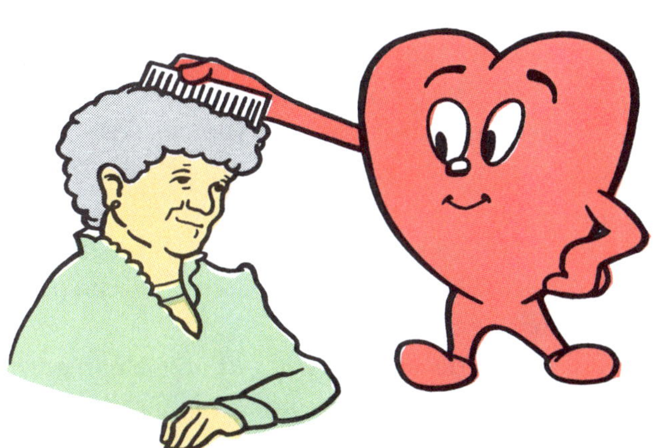

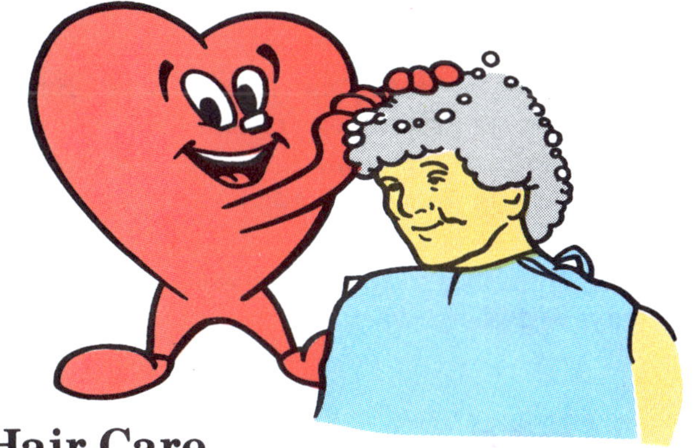

Hair Care

Daily Hair Care

Daily hair care includes brushing and combing. Be sure the patient's comb and brush are clean. Comb long, tangled hair one section at a time. Encourage patients to care for their own hair, if able.

Weekly Hair Care

Hair should be shampooed at least once a week.

1. Wash your hands.
2. Explain what you are going to do.
3. Assemble equipment:
   * mild shampoo
   * creme rinse
   * towel
   * comb or brush
4. Brush hair gently, removing tangles.
5. Adjust the water temperature for comfort.
6. Shampoo during showering, if permitted.
7. Wet the hair.
8. Shampoo gently, massaging the scalp.
9. Avoid getting soap in the patient's eyes.
10. Watch for scalp irritations or problems.
11. Use creme rinse if the patient desires it.
12. Rinse and dry:
    * towel (pat gently)
    * hair dryer
13. Style in a way the patient desires.
14. Make the patient comfortable.
15. Clean the equipment.
16. Wash your hands.
17. Report unusual observations to the supervisor.

If the facility has a beauty shop, remind the patient of his or her appointment. Help the patient to the shop if needed.

Bathing

Bathing provides more than cleanliness. Baths encourage exercise, stimulate circulation, prevent bedsores, promote relaxation, and give the NA an opportunity to spot problems such as infections or sores.

Encourage patients to wash themselves if they are able. Always provide privacy.

A.M. and P.M. Care

Every morning (a.m.) and every evening (p.m.) patients need care consisting of washing the face, back, armpits, and perineum. Gather all necessary equipment before you begin.

Perineal Care

Perineal care (or pericare) is cleansing of the genitalia and rectum. Pericare is given during the daily bath and after urinating or defecating.

Cleansing is always done from the front to the back, using warm water.

1. Gather equipment (see bed baths).

2. Wash your hands.

3. Explain what you are going to do.

4. Put on gloves.

5. With a mitted washcloth, separate the labia (female patient) with one hand and cleanse the area with downward strokes. Clean the penis (male patient) with circular motions. Pull back the foreskin of the uncircumcised male to clean the area.

6. Cover the area when finished.

7. Help the patient to a side-lying position.

8. Clean the rectum by wiping from the front to the back.

9. Make the patient comfortable.

10. Clean and store equipment.

11. Wash your hands.

12. Report any unusual odors, discharges, swelling, or redness.

Bed Baths

Full or partial bed baths are necessary for non-ambulatory patients. Encourage the patient to help as much as possible.

1. Assemble equipment:
   - towels
   - washcloth
   - bath blanket
   - soap
   - basin
   - clean gown
2. Identify the patient and explain what you are going to do.
3. Provide privacy, and close doors and windows to prevent drafts.
4. Offer toileting.
5. Adjust the bed to a comfortable position.
6. Remove the blankets, and place a bath blanket over the top sheet.
7. Remove the patient's gown and cover with a bath blanket.
8. Fill the basin two-thirds with warm water.
9. Help the patient move toward you.
10. Place a towel under the patient's farthest arm to keep the bed dry.
11. Make a mitt of the washcloth — fold in thirds around your hand, fold the top down, and tuck the bottom end under.
12. Wash the eyes from the inner to the outer corner, using water only, and rinse the cloth after each eye.
13. Wash and rinse the patient's face, neck, ears.
14. Dry well.
15. Work from the head down, washing with long, circular motions, washing, rinsing, and drying thoroughly.
16. Change the water frequently when it is soapy or cool.
17. If the patient is able, offer the washcloth for cleaning the perineal area.
18. Turn the patient to the side and place a towel on the bottom sheet by the patient's back.
19. Wash, rinse, and dry the backside.
20. Place the bath blanket under the legs, and bend the knees to wash and dry legs and feet.
21. When bathing is completed, give the patient a back rub.
22. Apply deodorant, and put on a clean gown.
23. Make the patient comfortable, raise the side rails, and place the call signal within reach.

Safety Guidelines

- Use extreme caution to prevent slips and falls.
- Test the water temperature, then have the patient test it.
- Always assist a patient in and out of the tub or shower.
- Never leave a patient alone while bathing.

Shower Bath

1. Assemble equipment:
   - towel
   - soap
   - washcloth
   - clean gown or clothes

2. Use a shower chair for safety so the patient does not have to stand for long periods.

3. Check the water temperature before the patient enters the shower.

4. Assist the patient into the shower.
   - Steady the ambulatory patient with your arm.
   - Make sure the wheelchair wheels are locked during transfer to the shower chair.

5. Assist as needed in washing, rinsing, drying, and dressing.

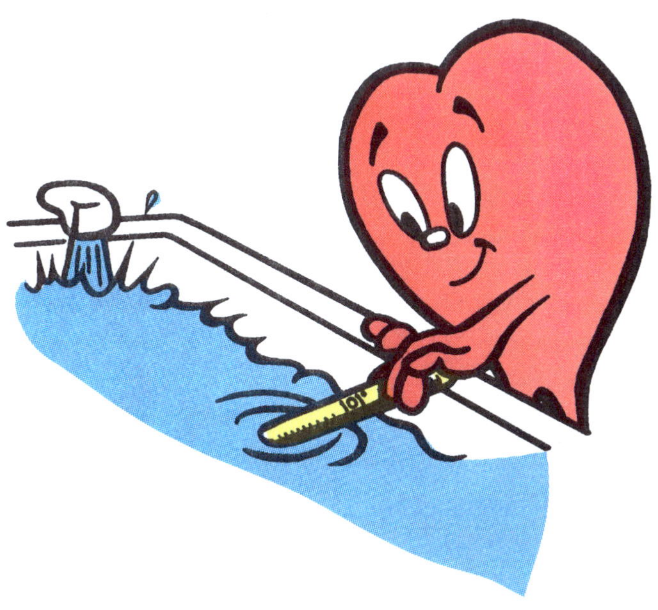

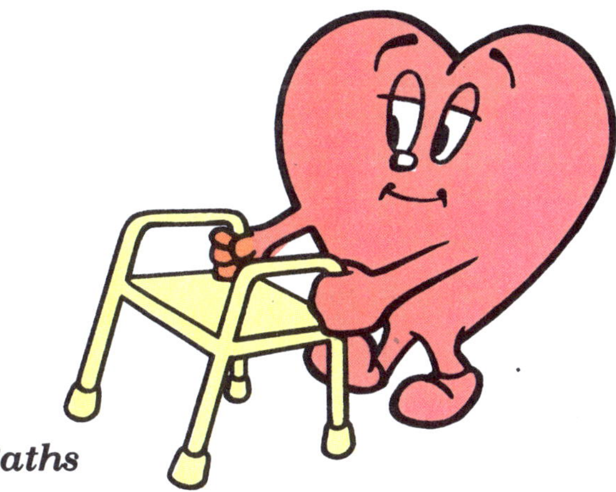

Tub Baths

1. Assemble the same equipment as a shower bath.

2. Fill the tub half full and test the water with a tub thermometer (101° - 105° F).

3. Make sure there are safety strips on the tub to prevent slipping.

4. Assist the patient into the tub.

5. Assist as needed in washing, rinsing, drying, and dressing.

Dressing

The NA helps patients who need assistance to dress and undress.

1. Tell the patient what you are going to do.
2. Wash your hands.
3. Help select clothes.
4. Prepare clothing by unbuttoning, unhooking, unzipping.
5. Provide privacy.
6. Gently remove clothing one area at a time, keeping the patient covered as much as possible.
7. Gently dress the patient:
   - Slacks: gather them at the leg, and reach through to guide the patient's ankle through.
   - Shirt or dress: gently pull the patient's hand through the sleeve.
   - Pullovers: gently guide both arms into the sleeves and slide the garment over the patient's head.
8. Smooth the clothing and fasten as needed.

Nail Care

The patient's nails should be short, smooth, and clean. Always check with your supervisor before giving nail care. Only a licensed nurse is allowed to trim the nails of diabetic patients.

Fingernails

1. Wash your hands.

2. Assemble equipment:
   - nail file
   - clippers
   - polish
   - basin of warm water
   - emery board
   - towel
   - lotion

3. Explain what you are going to do.

4. If nails are thick, soak them in warm water first.

5. Trim torn or rough edges.

6. Fingernails should be rounded.

7. Trim any hangnails carefully to prevent tearing.

8. Clean nails carefully with a nail file.

9. Smooth the edges with an emery board.

10. Encourage finger exercises and observe mobility.

11. Apply lotion.

12. Polish the nails if the patient desires.

13. Clean the equipment.

14. Remove and dispose of gloves.

15. Wash your hands.

Toenails

Procedures for foot care are the same as hand care with these exceptions:

- Check with the CN before giving nail care. Many patients (diabetics) require care by a podiatrist.

- Check for blisters, sores, corns, infections, or swelling.

- Toenails should be trimmed straight across.

- Clean and dry between and under toes.

- Report foot problems to your supervisor.

Shaving

Shaving is an individual choice. Many male patients prefer a clean-shaven face. Many women desire to shave their legs and underarms. Shave after bathing, when the skin is soft, or use a warm washcloth to soften the skin.

1. Wash your hands.

2. Gather equipment:
   - razor
   - towel
   - washcloth

3. Explain what you are going to do.

4. Help the patient to wash with warm water.

5. Apply shaving cream.

6. Hold the skin taut.

7. Shave in the direction the hair grows.

8. Apply after-shave lotion if desired.

9. Make the patient comfortable.

10. Clean equipment.

11. Wash your hands.

When using a patient's electric razor, be sure the area to be shaved is dry. Check that the razor has been cleaned with disinfectant between shavings. Observe precautions for using electrical equipment.

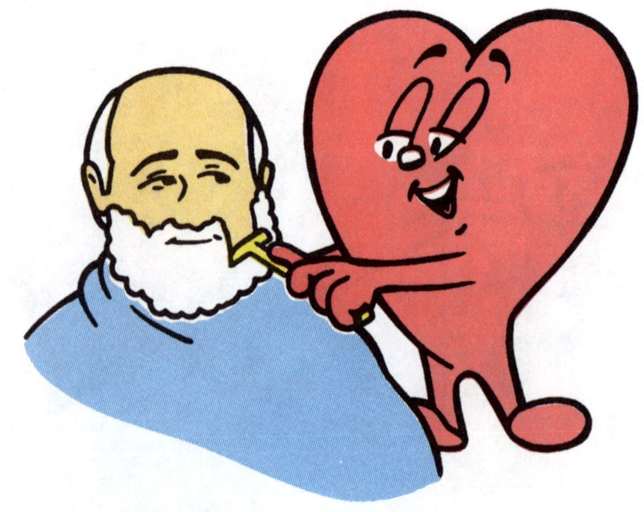

<table><tr><td>**Part 5**</td><td><h1>Serving Food</h1></td></tr></table>

Make mealtimes enjoyable for the patients.

Doctors recommend diets that are **therapeutic** (aid good health) for each patient. Dieticians prepare meals according to the doctor's orders.

> Always check the patient's diet order card with the meal being served. Serving the wrong meal could cause severe problems.

Encourage patients to go to the dining room for meals if possible. Dining with others provides an opportunity to socialize.

For patients who must eat in their rooms, take a few minutes to chat and make mealtime special. Provide assistance as needed. For patients who need extra help, check their care plans to find out if self-feeding programs have been developed.

Before Meals

Food service requires personal cleanliness.

- Wash your hands before and after serving food.
- Be sure your fingernails are clean.
- Clothing should be neat and clean.
- Long hair should be tied back.
- Keep your hands away from your face and mouth.
- Keep your fingers out of the food or beverages.
- Do not smoke.
- Protect any cuts with a waterproof bandage or use disposable gloves.

Before serving the food tray, check the patient's wrist identification, and ask the patient to tell you his or her name.

Correct: *"Please tell me your name."*

Incorrect: *"Are you Mrs. Smith?"*
(The patient may answer in error.)

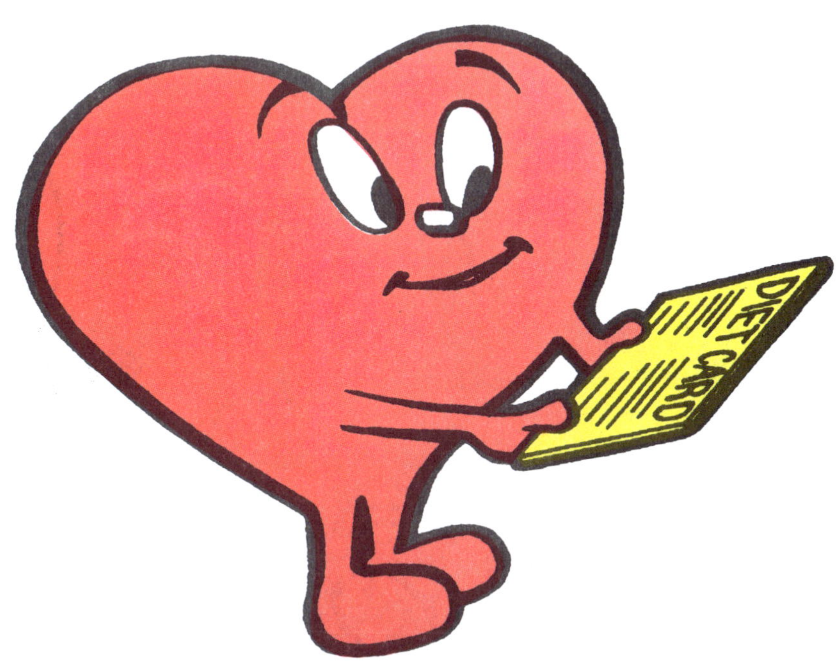

Serving Food

- Check the diet card and compare it with the meal you are serving to be sure it is the correct meal.
- Make sure the tray has proper silverware, food, napkins, beverages, and cup or straw. Pick up eating utensils with the handle.
- Assist with pouring drinks and cutting food as needed.
- Provide special eating utensils for patients who need them.

During Meals

- Be sure the patient is properly positioned for eating.
- Sit beside the patient at eye level.
- Carry on a pleasant conversation.
- Offer plenty of liquids, using a straw if the patient has trouble drinking from a cup (except for stroke patients).
- Feed the food slowly.
- Offer small amounts of food at a time.
- Allow time to chew and swallow.
- Watch for signs of gagging or choking!

Dysphagia (difficulty in swallowing) is a problem related to decreased saliva. If you observe a patient having difficulty swallowing, report it to your supervisor.

Feeding Tubes

Special tubes are sometimes used for patients who have difficulty swallowing. Tubes are ordered only by a doctor and placed by a licensed nurse. A nutritionally balanced liquid diet is fed through the tube using a pump.

The **nasogastric (ng)** tube is inserted into the patient's nostril and goes into the stomach.

The **gastric** tube is inserted directly through the abdominal wall.

The NA must be careful in moving, bathing, or dressing a patient with a nasogastric or gastric tube to avoid pulling on the tube.

- Report any signs of discomfort to the supervisor immediately.
- Watch for any irritation around the nostril.
- If the tube becomes blocked, report it immediately.
- Keep the head of the bed raised to 30 degrees.
- Keep all food and beverages away from patients whose orders indicate **nothing by mouth** (NPO).
- Always report any unusual observations.

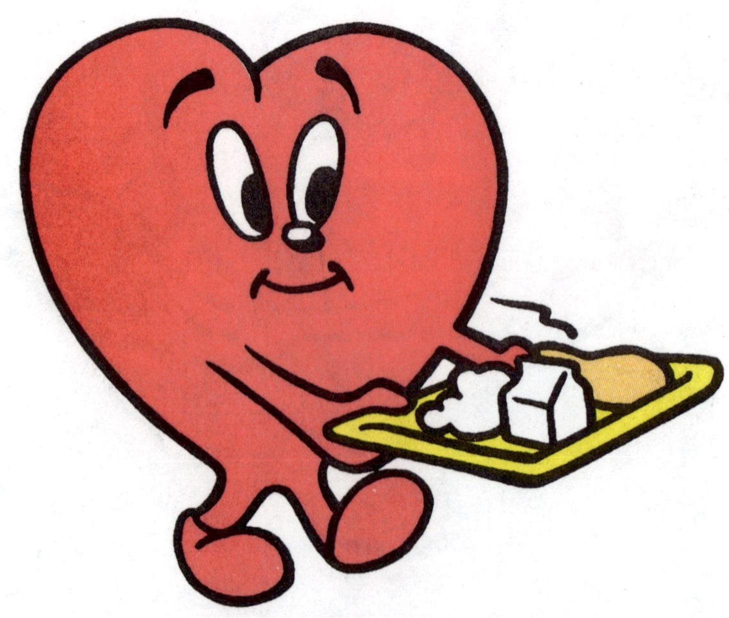

Part 6 — Weighing and Measuring

Changes in weight and height may indicate medical problems.

Patients are weighed and measured when admitted and periodically thereafter. Accuracy is important. Learn to use the scales in your facility safely and correctly.

The most commonly used scale is the standing-balance scale with a measuring rod. For patients who cannot stand, there are bed, wheelchair, and mechanical-lift scales.

Guidelines for weighing:

- **weigh at the same time of day**
- **wear the same weight of clothing**
- **weigh with an empty bladder**
- **remove footwear**

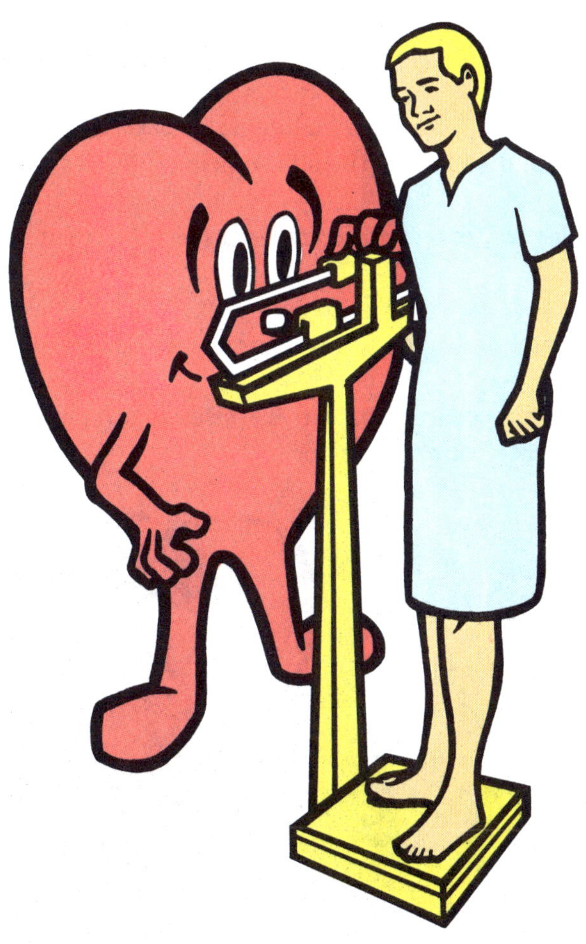

Weighing with the Standing-balance Scale

Using the standing-balance scale:

1. Explain what you are going to do.

2. Provide privacy.

3. Place both weights at zero with the balance centered.

4. Assist the patient onto the scale.

5. Be sure the patient is not holding onto you or the scale, and slide the bottom weight until the balance drops and centers.

6. Slide the top weight until the balance drops and centers.

7. Add the numbers shown at the weights.

8. Chart the weight.

Measuring with the Standing-balance Scale

1. To measure, place the rod above the patient's head.

2. Ask the person to turn away from the scale and stand straight.

3. Place the measuring rod against the top of the patient's head.

4. Read and record the patient's height.

5. Assist the patient in getting off the scale.

6. Report any major changes in height or weight.

Part 7 — Range of Motion (ROM)

*Encourage simple exercises at least three times a day
to help patients maintain mobility.*

Long periods of inactivity cause **contractures** (permanent shortening of muscles). Contractures are painful and limit use. They most commonly affect joints in the fingers, hands, elbows, knees, and hips.

Range-of-motion (ROM) exercises help increase the mobility of joints and prevent **atrophy** (wasting away) of muscle tissue.

Check each patient's care plan and follow the instructions carefully. ROM exercises should be done three or more times each day.

ROM Terms

Some terms the NA should know:

Abduction — moving a body part away from the body

Adduction — moving a body part toward the body

Extension — straightening a body part

Flexion — bending a body part

Hyperextension — excessive straightening

Dorsal Flexion — bending backward

Rotation — turning a joint
    Internal — turning inward
    External — turning outward

Pronation — turning downward

Supination — turning upward

Perform ROM exercises only as directed. Begin with the head and work down to the feet. Exercise one side of the body at a time, working each joint through the normal range of movement. Encourage patients to perform the exercises by themselves if they can.

Plan your day to combine tasks whenever possible. For example, a patient who does self-oral care also completes range-of-motion exercises for the arm. As you observe and encourage movement throughout the day, do ROM exercises at the same time.

Performing ROM Exercises

- Support the joint and move it gently and smoothly through its normal range three to five times.

- Move joints slowly.

- If a joint is red or swollen, do not exercise it until directed by the supervisor.

- Never force a joint or move it past the point of pain.

- Watch the patient's face for signs of pain.

- If pain occurs, stop the exercises and report the pain to your supervisor.

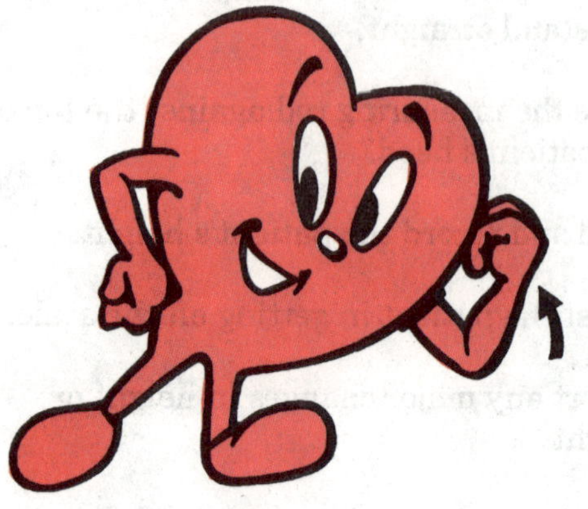

Flexion

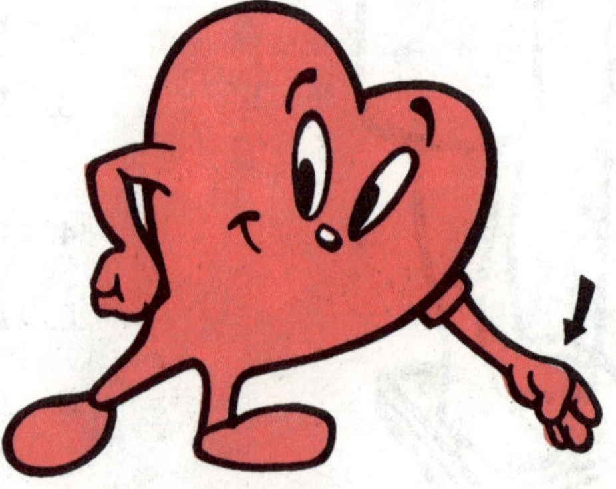

Extension

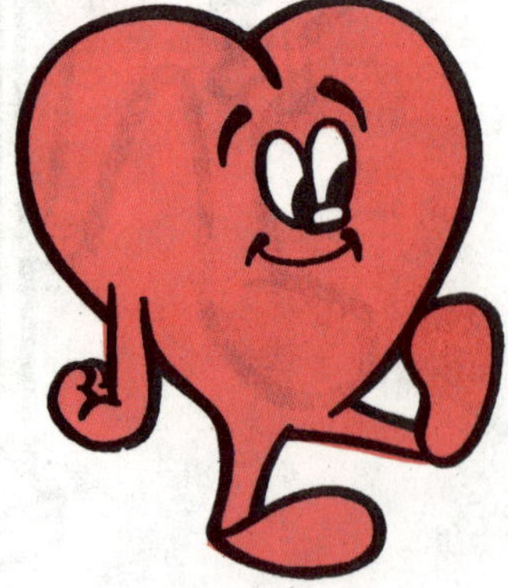

Dorsal Flexion

Part 8 — Giving a Back Rub

Back rubs help relieve tension and increase circulation.

Back rubs are usually given in the morning after the patient has bathed. They may be part of evening care to relax the patient or for patients requiring special skin care.

1. Gather equipment:
   - towel
   - lotion
   - basin of warm water

2. Wash your hands.

3. Provide privacy.

4. Explain what you are going to do.

5. Warm the lotion in the basin of water.

6. Ask the patient to turn his or her back toward you, assisting as needed.

7. Lay the towel lengthwise on the bed behind the patient's back.

8. Apply the lotion with long, firm strokes. Move from the buttocks to the back of the neck.

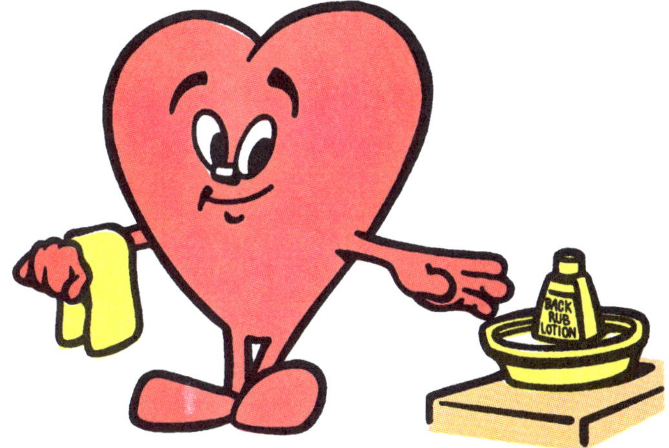

9. Use firm pressure when stroking upward and gentle pressure when stroking downward.

10. Rub the bony areas with a circular motion.

11. Rub the back for approximately three minutes.

12. Pat the back dry with a towel.

13. Make the patient comfortable.

14. Replace the side rails.

15. Wash your hands.

16. Chart the procedure.

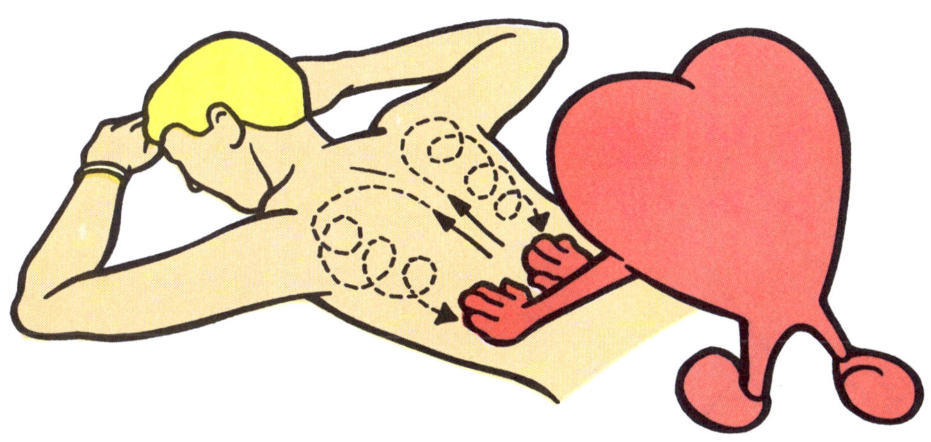

NA Review

1. Explain why careful observation is important.

2. Describe how to correct a chart entry.

3. How can the NA promote independence?

4. Describe three safety precautions when assisting patients in bathing.

1.) Test the water temperatures.

5. Why is proper bed making important?

6. Explain an important safety precaution in making an occupied bed.

7. What is ROM, and why is it important?

8. When would the NA **not** give nail care, and how do you determine this?

Vocabulary

abduction	(ab-**duck**-shun)	moving body part away from body
adduction	(a-**duck**-shun)	moving body part toward body
aspiration	(as-pi-**ray**-shun)	breathing in solids or fluids
atrophy	(**at**-ruh-fee)	wasting away of muscle or other tissue
dentures	(**den**-churz)	false teeth
dysphagia	(dis-**fay**-jee-ah)	difficulty swallowing
hygiene	(**hy**-jeen)	science of cleanliness and health
nasogastric	(nay-zo-**gas**-trick)	soft plastic tube inserted through nostril into stomach
objective	(ob-**jeck**-tiv)	reporting facts
perineal	(per-i-**nee**-ul)	rectal and genital areas
rehabilitate	(re-hah-**bil**-i-tate)	restore what has been lost
subjective	(sub-**jeck**-tiv)	giving an opinion

Additional Terms to Remember

____

____

____

____

____

____

____

____

____

NA Notes

Promote independence by assisting patients only as needed.

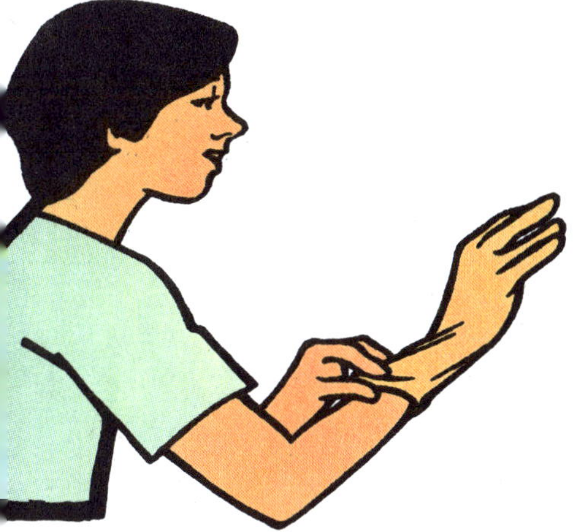

Elimination

Objectives:

- ☐ Describe toileting procedures
- ☐ Explain how to measure intake and output (I/O)
- ☐ Demonstrate urine tests
- ☐ Describe patient care for an indwelling catheter
- ☐ Explain bowel and bladder training techniques
- ☐ Describe the procedure for giving an enema

Part 1 — Using Bedpans

Provide privacy and minimize the patient's anxiety.

Elimination is the body's natural process for getting rid of wastes and is essential for the body to function. The patient who needs help may be embarrassed. It is the NA's job to be professional, provide privacy, and minimize the patient's anxiety.

If the patient is unable to use the bathroom toilet, provide alternatives.

Bedpans

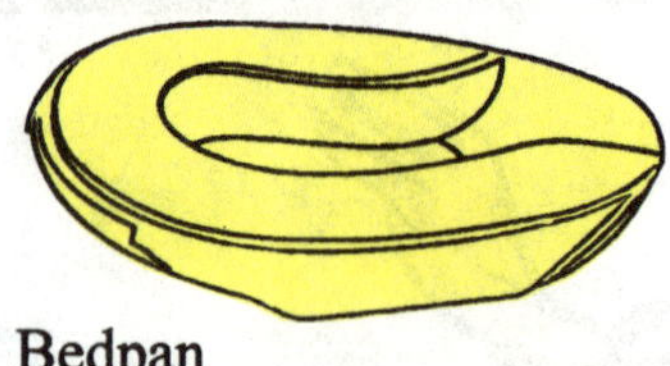

Bedpan

Bedpan

for women: to **void** (urinate)
                to **defecate** (bowel movement)

for men: to defecate

Urinal

for men: to void

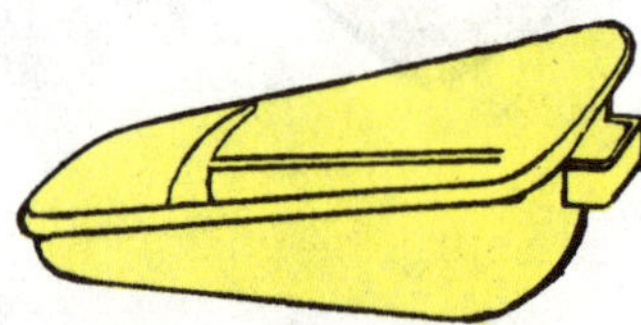

Fracture pan

Fracture pan

for patients with hip fractures

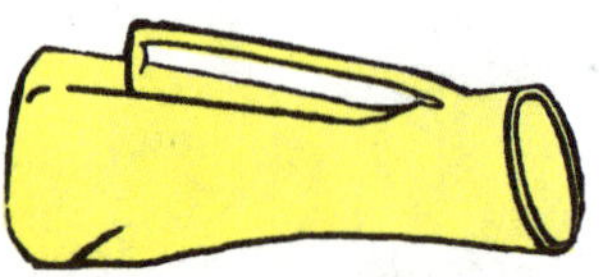

Urinal

Procedure

1. Wash your hands.
2. Put on gloves.
3. Assemble equipment:
   - washcloth
   - toilet
   - pan and cover
   - towel
4. Provide privacy.
5. Pre-warm the bedpan if necessary.
6. Ask the patient to bend his or her knees with feet flat on the bed and raise the hips. Assist if needed with your hand under the patient's lower back.
7. Place the pan.
8. If the patient is unable to raise the hips, roll him or her away from you, place the pan, and roll the patient onto the pan.
9. Raise the patient to a sitting position if possible.
10. Cover the patient with a sheet.
11. Raise the bed rails.
12. Place the toilet tissue and the call light within easy reach.
13. Ask the patient to signal when done.
14. Never leave a patient on a bedpan for more than 10 minutes. (Within 10 minutes check whether the patient needs assistance.)

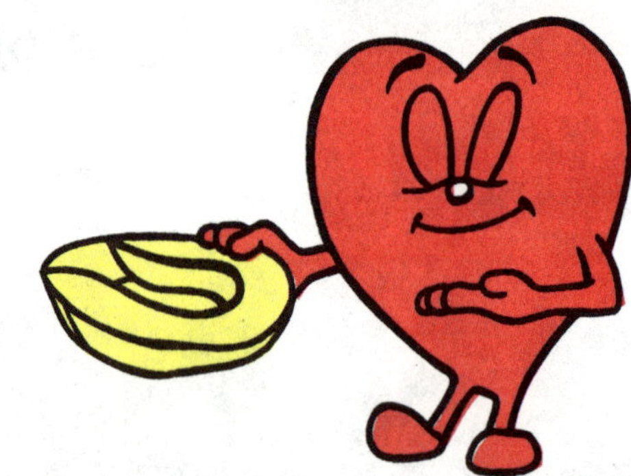

15. Remove the bedpan and cover it immediately.
16. Assist with wiping and hand washing as needed.
17. Take the pan to the bathroom.
18. Collect a specimen or measurement of output if needed.
19. Dispose of waste matter.
20. Remove and dispose of gloves.
21. Wash your hands.
22. Wash the pan in bacterial cleanser, dry thoroughly, and store in a clean bag in the patient's cupboard.

Bedside Commode

Some patients have the ability to get out of bed, but cannot use the bathroom. For those patients, there is a bedside **commode**.

The commode is a chair with a hole in the seat and a bedpan below. It is used like a toilet, but the pan must be removed and emptied after each use.

Procedure

1. Wash your hands.
2. Assemble equipment:
   - washcloth
   - towel
   - toilet tissue
   - bedpan

3. Make sure the bedpan or bucket is in the commode.

4. Provide privacy.
5. Explain the procedure to the patient.
6. Help the patient move to the commode.
7. Wash your hands and leave the room.
8. Respond to the call light quickly.
9. Put on gloves.
10. Assist with wiping and hand washing as needed.
11. Help the patient get into bed.

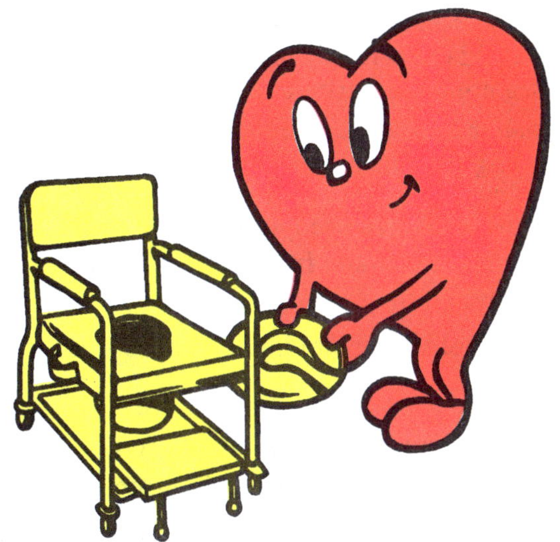

12. Cover and remove the bedpan.
13. Observe **feces** (waste matter) for blood or other problems.
14. Report any irregularities to your supervisor.
15. Clean the bedpan and store it.
16. Remove and dispose of gloves.
17. Wash your hands.

Part 2 Documenting Fluid Intake and Output (I/O)

Fluid balance is extremely important to good health.

The doctor or nurse may request a patient's **intake/output** (I/O) to be documented. This means recording the amount of fluids taken in and eliminated each day.

Edema (too much fluid in the tissues) may cause painful swelling and weight gain. Heart and kidney disease, as well as too much salt, can cause edema.

Some ways the NA can help make the patient with edema more comfortable:

- Encourage the patient to wear loose-fitting clothing.
- Raise the **extremity** (limb), using a stool or pillow.

Dehydration (too little fluid) may cause weight loss, dry and cracking skin, fever, constipation, and difficulty in swallowing.

Help prevent dehydration by encouraging the person to drink fluids.

- Always keep fresh water at the bedside, within easy reach.

- Offer to pour a drink for the patient when you enter the room (water, tea, coffee, juices).

- Offer foods such as gelatin, ice cream, or custard if the patient's diet allows them.

Measuring Intake

To get an accurate measurement of intake, it is necessary to record all fluids taken by the patient. Measure fluids taken by mouth as well as soft foods such as ice cream, gelatin, or custard.

Licensed nursing staff record **intravenous** (IV) fluids and ng tube feedings.

- Record intake as soon as it is consumed.
- Record water taken from bedside water pitchers.
- Record between-meal liquid snacks (coffee, tea, or juice).

Fluid measurements are recorded in **cubic centimeters** (cc). Make sure you know how much the containers hold and how to convert fluid measurements. One ounce = 30 cc. Most facilities provide conversion tables for measuring I/O.

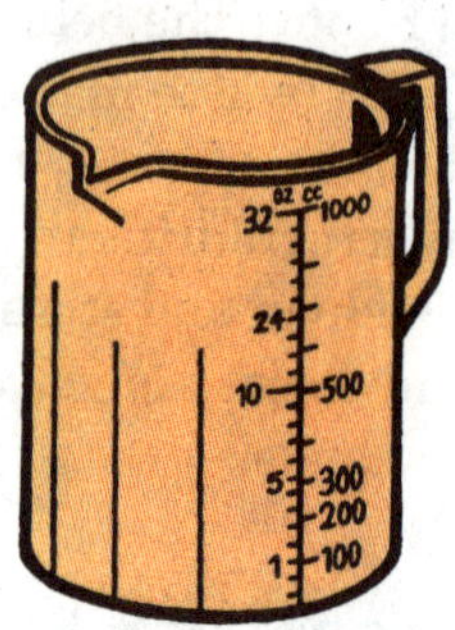

Measuring Output

Urine is the easiest and most reliable output measurement. For the ambulatory patient, a specimen pan is placed on the toilet seat. Ask the patient not to empty the pan. For patients using a bedpan, urinal, or commode, the NA removes the sample to the bathroom.

1. Wash your hands.
2. Put on gloves.
3. Pour the urine into a graduated specimen container.
4. Put the container on a level surface and note the output. Accuracy is extremely important.
5. Look for unusual observations in the urine:
   - blood
   - unusual odor or color
   - discharges
   - mucus
6. Empty the urine into the toilet and flush.
7. Remove and dispose of the gloves.
8. Record the output.
9. Clean all equipment.
10. Wash your hands.
11. Report any irregularities.

On the average, a person voids 1200 - 1500 cc per day.

Treating Bowel and Bladder Problems

Bladder and bowel problems need special attention.

Testing Urine

Observe urine for color, odor, amount, clarity, and frequency. Report any complaints the patient has.

Two urine tests you may be asked to do are the **clinitest** for sugar and the **acetest** for acetone.

1. Collect a fresh urine specimen from the patient.

2. Put on gloves.

3. Pour a small amount of urine into a glass test tube.

4. Dip the test strip into the urine.

5. Wait 15 seconds for the acetone test, then compare the strip to the color chart on the container for acetone.

6. Wait another 15 seconds, then compare to the color chart for sugar.

7. Dispose of used strips and flush the urine.

8. Remove and dispose of the gloves.

9. Wash your hands.

10. Clean and store all equipment.

Catheter Care

Patients who have difficulty urinating may have a **catheter** (sterile plastic tube) inserted. An **indwelling** (or Foley) **catheter** remains in the bladder and is connected to a drainage bag. Special catheter care is required daily to prevent infection.

1. Assemble equipment:
   - catheter care kit
   - disposable gloves
   - bed protector

2. Wash your hands.

3. Provide privacy.

4. Tell the patient what you are going to do.

5. Ask the patient to bend the knees; and, with feet flat on the bed, raise the buttocks. Place the bed protector under the patient.

6. Drape the patient.

7. Put on gloves.

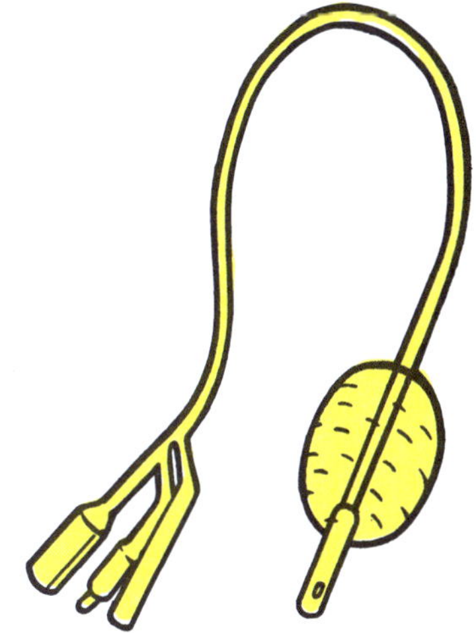

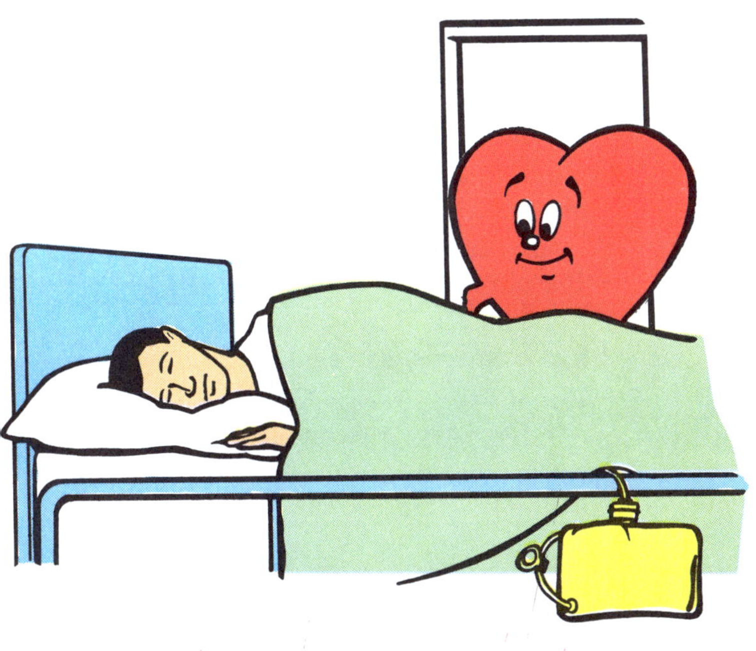

8. Provide perineal care.

9. Open the catheter kit.

10. Open the antiseptic packet.

11. Check the labia (females) or foreskin (males) for crusts, sores, bleeding, or leakage. Report any problems to your supervisor immediately.

12. Apply antiseptic to the labia (women) or head of the penis (men), using a new applicator for each stroke.

13. Use a fresh antiseptic pad to clean the first four inches of the catheter tubing, starting nearest the patient and wiping toward you.

14. Inspect the tubing for cracks, kinks, or leaks.

15. Discard the bed protector and antiseptic pads.

16. Remove and discard the gloves.

17. Cover the patient and position for comfort.

18. Raise the side rail and place the call signal within reach.

19. Clean the area.

20. Wash your hands.

Bowel and Bladder Training

Training programs can help patients regain control of elimination. If a training plan has been established, follow the instructions carefully.

Incontinence is the lack of ability to control the bladder and/or bowels. The NA's reaction is very important. Never embarrass or scold the patient. Keep the patient clean and dry, and give perineal care promptly.

Help the patient regain control:

- Provide frequent toileting.

- Encourage plenty of fluids — 2000 to 2500 cc per day.

- Keep accurate records of intake and output.

- Praise the patient who is making progress. (Never scold a patient for an "accident.")

Bowel movements vary from person to person and are affected by medications, diet, fluids, and activity. It is important to observe the frequency, amount, color, odor, and texture of the stools. Report any problems related to bowel elimination.

Constipation is bowel elimination that is infrequent and painful with hard feces. Care includes adjusting the diet, increasing fluids, and more activity. If these measures are not effective, a suppository or enema may be ordered.

Impaction is the inability to pass **stools** (feces). Report symptoms of impaction immediately:

- pain in the abdomen or rectum

- small amounts of liquid seeping from the anus

- the urge to defecate, but cannot

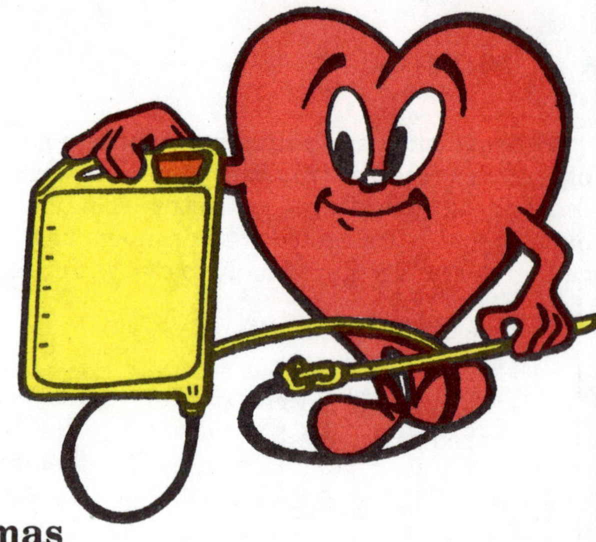

Enemas

An enema introduces liquid into the rectum. Enemas are ordered by the doctor to relieve constipation or to clean the bowel prior to special procedures.

Procedure

1. Wash your hands.

2. Assemble equipment:
   - bedpan or commode
   - bath thermometer
   - toilet tissue
   - waterproof bed protector
   - enema kit
   - lubricant
   - bath blanket

3. Put on gloves.

4. Provide privacy.

5. Explain what you are going to do.

6. Prepare the enema:
   - For tap water, add nothing to the water.
   - For saline, add two teaspoons of salt.
   - For soap suds, add 5 ml of liquid soap.

7. Check the water temperature ($105°$).

8. Clamp the tubing.

9. Position the patient in the left Sim's position.

10. Cover the patient with the bath blanket to expose the anal area.

11. Place the waterproof bed protector under the buttocks.

12. Place the bedpan behind the patient.

13. Unclamp the tubing and allow enough solution to flow into the bedpan to remove air from the tubing.

14. Ask the patient to take a deep breath through the mouth.

15. As the patient exhales, gently insert the tubing two to four inches into the rectum.

16. Stop if the patient complains of discomfort or you feel resistance. Do not force the tubing.

17. Continue the enema until the ordered amount has been given, the patient can no longer tolerate the procedure, or the patient expresses a desire to defecate.

18. Clamp the tubing before the enema bag is empty to prevent air from entering the rectum.

19. Gently withdraw the tubing from the rectum.

20. Wrap the tip of the tubing with toilet tissue and place inside the enema bag.

21. Remove and discard gloves.

22. Help the patient onto the bedpan, commode, or toilet.

23. Place the toilet tissue and call light within easy reach.

24. Wash your hands and leave the room.

25. Answer the call light quickly.

26. Assist the patient with wiping and hand washing, if needed.

27. Help the patient to bed.

28. Clean up equipment.

29. Make the patient comfortable and replace side rails before leaving the room.

30. Wash your hands.

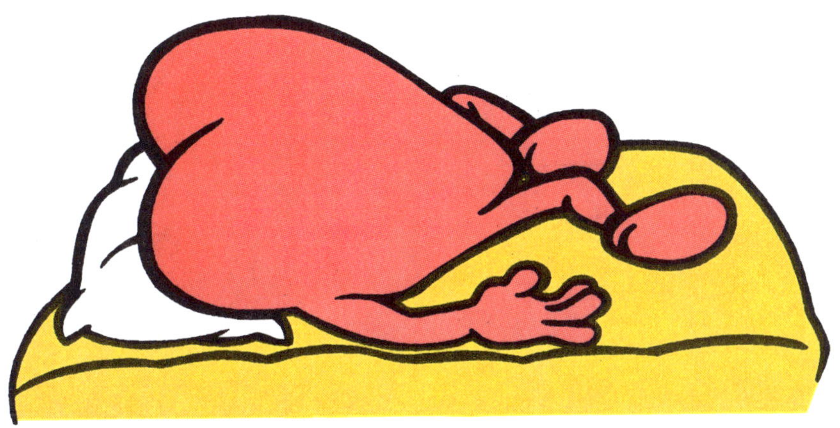

NA Review

1. Explain the use of bedpans, urinals, fracture pans, and bedside commodes.

2. What is dehydration, and how can the NA prevent it?

3. Identify five observations for urine.

1) Frequency

4. Describe catheter care.

5. Explain bowel and bladder training programs.

6. Who orders enemas, and why?

Vocabulary

catheter	(**kath**-e-ter)	plastic drain tube for bladder
commode	(kom-**mod**)	bedside chair containing bedpan
constipation	(kon-sti-**pay**-shun)	difficult bowel movement
defecate	(**def**-e-kate)	bowel movement
dehydration	(dee-hy-**dray**-shun)	too little fluid in body tissues
edema	(e-**dee**-mah)	too much fluid in tissues
enema	(**en**-e-mah)	injecting liquid into rectum
feces	(**fee**-seez)	body waste from the bowels
impaction	(im-**pack**-shun)	inability to pass feces
incontinence	(in-**kon**-ti-nens)	lack of control of bladder and/or bowel
intravenous	(in-truh-**vee**-nus)	directly into vein

Additional Terms to Remember

____

____

____

____

____

____

____

____

____

____

____

NA Notes

Provide privacy and never embarrass the patient.

Lesson 8

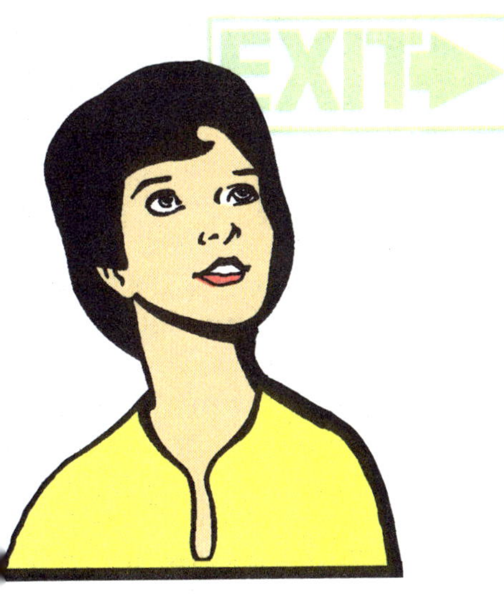

Safety and Emergency Procedures

Protect your patients from life-threatening injuries!

Objectives:

- ☐ Discuss accident prevention
- ☐ Demonstrate the Heimlich Maneuver
- ☐ Explain CPR procedures
- ☐ Identify fire hazards
- ☐ Demonstrate emergency procedures in case of fire
- ☐ Demonstrate the use of restraints and safety devices

<table><tr><td>**Part 1**</td><td># Preventing Accidents</td></tr></table>

The best way to avoid an accident is to be alert to potential hazards!

Some simple precautions can prevent serious injuries.

Preventing Falls and Bruises

- Remove obstacles to walking such as personal belongings, cords, or equipment.
- Wipe up spills immediately.
- Do not leave a helpless patient unattended.
- Assist patients in and out of the bath.
- Use proper lighting.
- Lock wheels when moving patients to and from wheelchairs or gurneys.
- Keep items that are used frequently close at hand so the patient won't fall reaching for them.
- Answer the call light promptly so the patient won't try to get up.
- Encourage patients to use handrails when walking.
- Assist patients with walking if needed.
- Be alert to furniture or objects that pose a hazard.
- When moving a wheelchair, do not let the patient's feet drag on the floor.
- Be cautious in the use of restraints.

Preventing Burns

Cigarettes: prevent burns by enforcing safe smoking procedures.

Bath Water: make sure the water is not too hot. Test the water, and then have the patient test the water.

K-pads: use moisture-heated pads in place of hot water bottles and heating pads.

Hot Liquids: assist patients with hot foods and liquids.

Accidental Poisoning

Keep all cleansers and disinfectants locked in proper storage areas.

Choking

- Encourage patients to eat slowly, taking small bites.
- Be sure the patient is positioned properly for eating and swallowing.

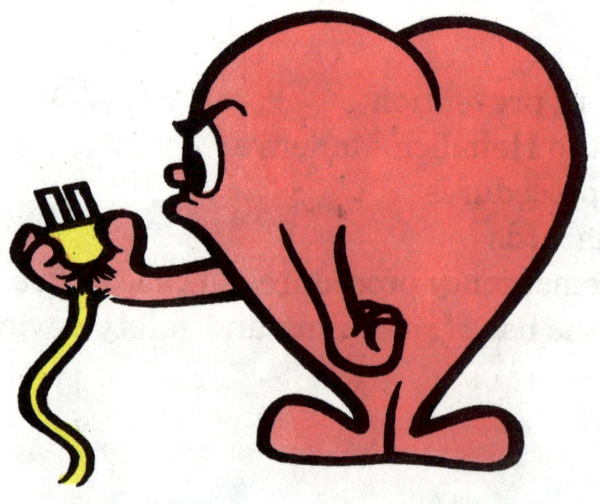

Preventing Electrical Shock

- Inspect all equipment for damage (such as frayed cords).
- Operate equipment according to instructions. If in doubt, ask.
- Always use properly grounded equipment.
- Be sure people and areas are dry before plugging in equipment.
- Do not overload circuits.
- Do not use extension cords.

 # Responding to Emergencies

Save lives by responding quickly.

Emergencies happen. Someone's life may depend on you, and you must act *fast!*

The Heimlich Maneuver

The Heimlich Maneuver is a first-aid procedure for choking. It is used only when there is a complete **obstruction** (blockage) of the airway.

Clutching the throat is the universal sign for choking. In case of choking, ask the patient to speak or cough. If the patient cannot speak or cough, or the response is very weak, proceed with the Heimlich Maneuver.

Procedure

1. Stand behind the patient.

2. Slide your arms under the victim's arms and wrap them around the waist.

3. Make a fist and place it against the person's abdomen, below the rib cage and above the navel, being careful not to touch the **sternum** (breastbone where the rib cage meets).

4. Using your free hand, apply pressure against your fist with an inward and upward thrust.

5. Give four rapid thrusts.

6. Repeat the procedure if necessary.

The abdominal thrusts dislodge the food and force it upward, out of the throat.

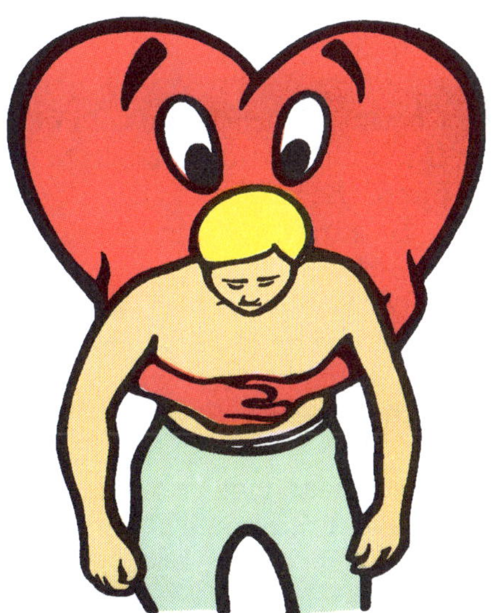

Treating an Unconscious Patient

If the person loses consciousness from choking, the neck muscles may relax enough that the object no longer completely obstructs the airway. You may be able to remove the obstruction.

If the airway is still blocked, use the following procedures:

1. Call for emergency help.

2. Place the patient on his or her back.

3. Open the airway by tilting the head back and lifting the chin.

4. Check for breath.

5. If there is no breath, open the mouth and try to sweep the mouth with your finger to remove the blockage (use a scooping motion rather than pulling).

6. Pinch the nose closed and **ventilate** (give air) with two full breaths.

7. If the airway is still blocked, kneel beside or straddle the patient at hip level.

8. Place the heel of your hand on the patient's abdomen below the rib cage with your fingers pointing toward the patient's chest.

9. Place your free hand over the positioned hand.

10. Place your shoulders over the patient's abdomen and press your hands inward and upward.

11. Give six to ten rapid thrusts.

12. Check to see if the obstruction is dislodged.

13. Try to sweep the object out with your scooped fingers.

14. Repeat steps 6 through 11 if necessary.

Cardiopulmonary Resuscitation (CPR)

CPR training teaches valuable life-saving skills, using mouth-to-mouth resuscitation and chest compression when the heart and/or lungs have stopped working. Only fully-trained people should administer CPR. If you have not already had a course in CPR, check with your instructor for classes in your area.

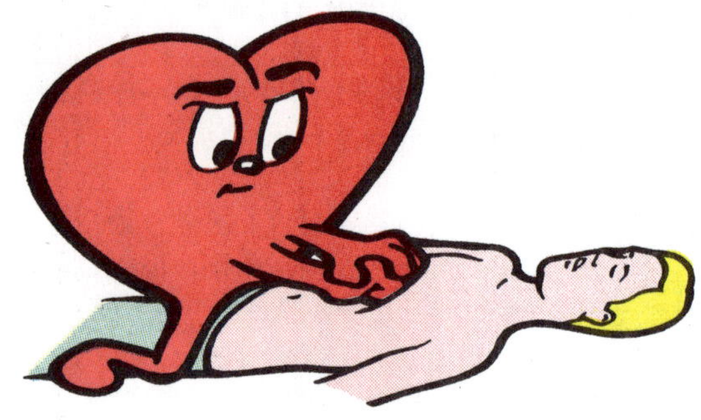

Quick action is critical. CPR is first-aid emergency care until medical help arrives. CPR must begin as soon as the heart stops in order to prevent brain and organ damage.

The following information is not a CPR course. It is intended as a basic review for those who have completed CPR training.

1. Call for help.

2. Shake the victim (unless you suspect a spinal injury) and call the person's name.

3. If there is no response, check for breathing.
   - **Look:** for chest movement
   - **Listen:** by putting your ear near the victim's nose and mouth
   - **Feel:** for breath on your cheek

4. If there is no breath, begin artificial respiration (you artificially breathe for the patient).

5. Use universal precautions to prevent infection. (Remember you are at risk with all patients.)

6. Tilt the head back by lifting the neck.

7. Check for any obstruction to the airway, and clear the airway if there is any blockage.

8. Pinch the nose closed to prevent air from escaping through the nostrils, and cover the victim's mouth completely with your mouth.

9. Blow into the person's mouth until you see the chest rise.
   - Blow two full breaths, and turn your head to the side to listen for air.

10. Check the carotid pulse (5 to 10 seconds). If there is no pulse, begin to artificially pump the victim's heart.
    - Be sure the victim is lying flat on a hard surface.
    - Locate the victim's sternum.
    - Lace your fingers together.
    - Use the heels of your hands to compress the chest 15 times.

11. Continue to give two breaths followed by 15 thrusts until medical help arrives.

<table><tr><td>Part 3</td><td># Fire Safety</td></tr></table>

Patients depend on you for their safety.

Fire can be a panic situation for a patient who is confined to a wheelchair or bed, or who has reduced mobility.

> In case of an emergency, stay calm and take immediate action to remove patients from danger.

Recognizing Hazards

Awareness of fire hazards is the first step toward prevention. Three elements are needed to start a fire. By removing any of these elements, a fire can be prevented:

heat:	flame or spark
oxygen:	normal air
fuel:	any **combustible material** (items that catch fire and burn easily)

Alert your supervisor if you smell smoke or if a door feels hot. **Do not open the door!**

Smoking

Never leave smoking patients unattended. Some patients may not be able to handle smoking materials safely because of medications or reduced abilities.

Smoking materials should be stored for safekeeping.

Strictly follow the facility's smoking policy.

- Smoking is allowed in authorized areas only.
- Use noncombustible ashtrays.
- Empty ashtrays into "butt cans" (metal containers partially filled with sand).
- **Never permit smoking where oxygen is in use.**
- Never use paper cups or trash cans for ashtrays.

Storage

Never store oily rags, paint cans, chemicals, or other combustibles in closed areas.

Faulty Wiring or Equipment

Inspect all equipment that you use and report any defects. Do not use faulty equipment:

- frayed power cords
- overloaded circuits
- overheated equipment
- improperly grounded equipment

Aerosol Cans

Never burn aerosol cans. Never use aerosol spray near open flames or cigarettes.

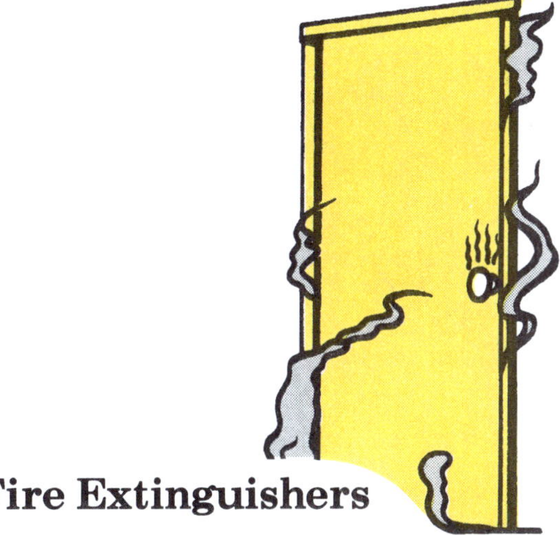

Fire Extinguishers

Different types of extinguishers are used for different types of fires. Be sure you have the proper extinguisher for the fire!

Oil and grease fires: Use a dry chemical extinguisher. Never use water on oil or grease.

Electrical fires: Use a multipurpose extinguisher. Never use water.

Paper and wood fires: Use a water extinguisher.

Emergency Procedures

Be sure you know the facility's emergency procedures:

- Understand fire and evacuation procedures.
- Know the location of all exits.
- Know where the fire alarms and extinguishers are located.

In case of fire, remember **RACE!**
- **R** — rescue
- **A** — alarm
- **C** — contain
- **E** — extinguish

1. **Rescue** any patients in immediate danger.

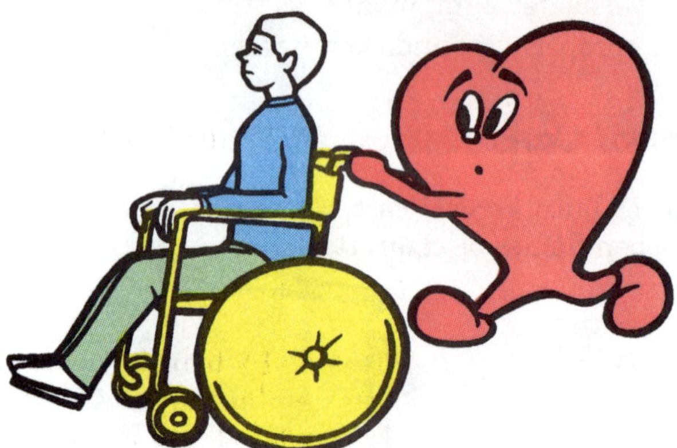

2. Sound the **alarm.**

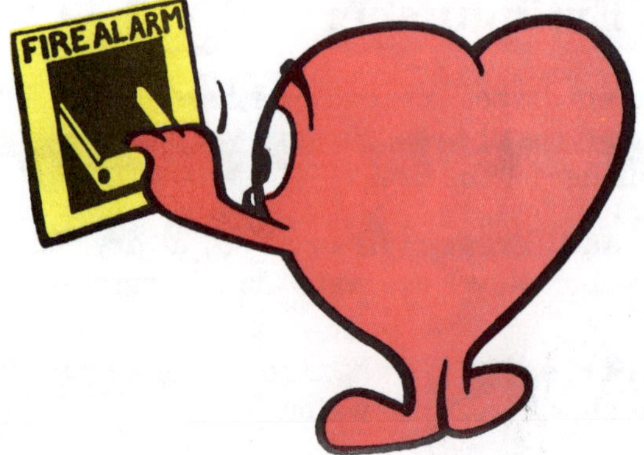

3. **Contain** the fire by closing doors and windows.

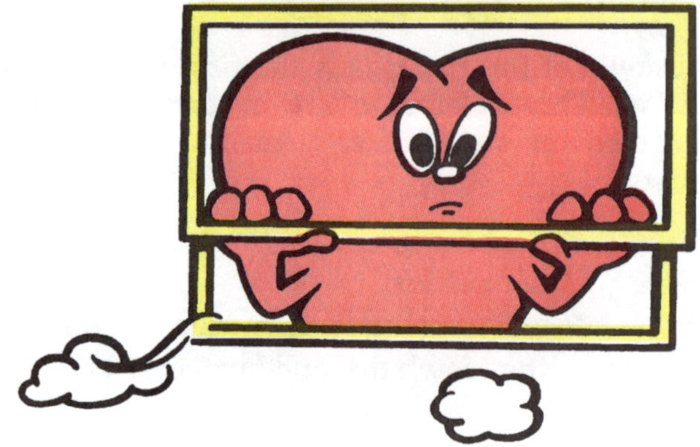

4. **Extinguish** the fire, if possible, using the proper extinguisher.

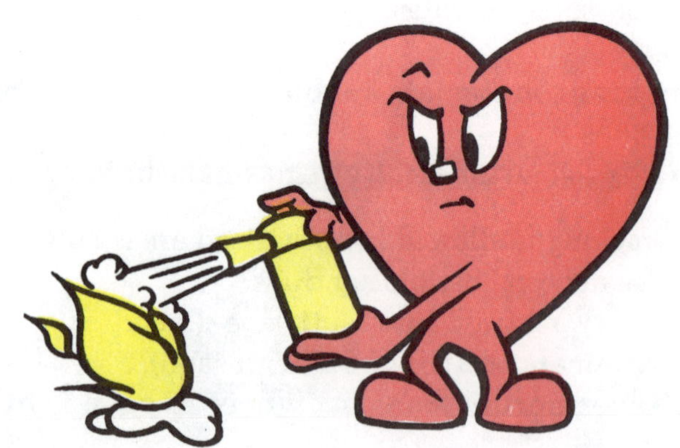

<table><tr><td>Part 4</td><td># Using Protective Devices</td></tr></table>

Restraints require a doctor's written orders.

Restraints (protective devices) infringe on the patient's rights by limiting movement. They are used to protect patients from harm when other methods have failed.

Restraints require a doctor's written orders that specify a specific type of protective device, length of time, and purpose for using the device. Neither physical nor chemical restraints are used for discipline or convenience. Legal charges may be filed if restraints are used unnecessarily.

Protective devices include safety belts, limb ties, jackets, vests, mitts, and pelvic supports. They limit movement of the chest, waist, elbows, ankles, wrists, or fingers and provide:

- support and comfort
- safety
- protection from injury to self or others
- limited movement of treatment supplies (IV tubes, etc.)
- healing

Applying Restraints

1. Tell the patient why you are applying the device.

2. Tie snugly, without cutting off circulation. Check to be sure you can slip your fingers under the device after tying.

3. Pad the device to avoid discomfort to joints and skin.

4. Position the patient to protect from the discomfort of knots and buckles.

5. Straighten wrinkled clothing or linens.

6. Always position a call light within easy reach.

7. Make the patient comfortable and provide activity to stimulate circulation (reposition, massage, ROM, ambulate).

8. Check the patient frequently to be sure the device will not tighten or slip with movement. Observe the patient's color, circulation, respirations, and pulse. Report any problems immediately.

9. Carefully document the use of protective devices.

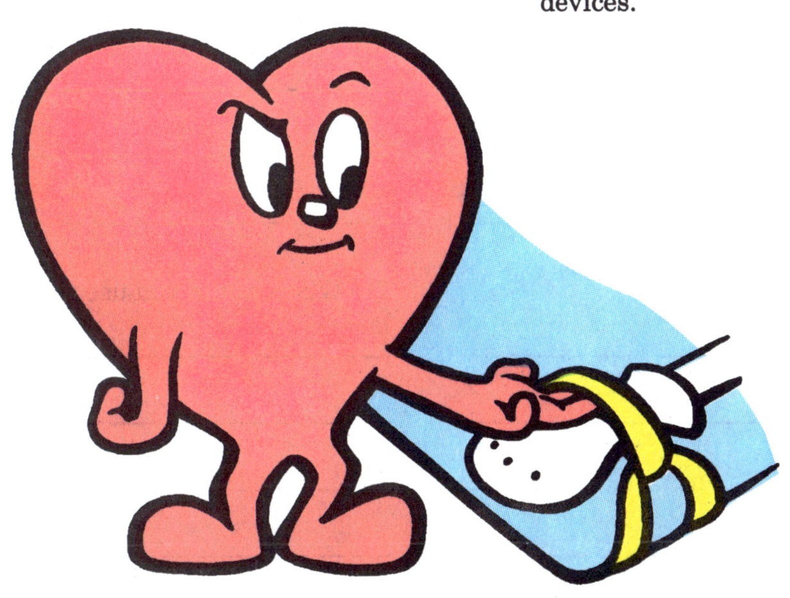

NA Review

1. Identify six or more ways to prevent falls.

   1) Wipe up spills immediately.

2. How can you prevent accidental poisoning?

3. Describe potential safety hazards.

4. What would you do in case of fire?

5. When would you use restraints and why?

6. Explain the Heimlich Maneuver and when you would use it.

7. When would you use CPR?

Vocabulary

cardiopulmonary resuscitation	(kar-de-o-**pull**-mo-ner-ee re-sus-i-**tay**-shun)	giving respiration and/or heart massage to revive a person
combustible	(kom-**bus**-ti-bul)	any material that will ignite or burn easily
obstruction	(ob-**struck**-shun)	blockage of airway or blood vessel
restraint	(re-**straynt**)	protective device that limits body movement

Additional Terms to Remember

____

____

____

____

____

____

____

____

____

____

____

____

____

____

NA Notes

Use of restraints must be carefully documented.

Lesson 9

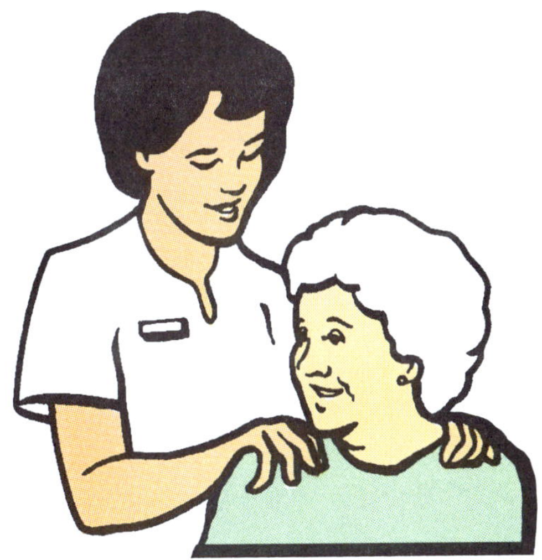

Specific Disorders

Your patience and support enhance the patient's quality of life!

Objectives:

- ☐ Demonstrate reality orientation
- ☐ Explain mental retardation
- ☐ Describe three phases of Alzheimer's Disease
- ☐ Recognize side effects of cancer treatment
- ☐ Identify the symptoms of diabetes
- ☐ Describe care of the patient with a pacemaker
- ☐ Discuss the steps to take during a seizure
- ☐ Identify effects of a stroke
- ☐ Recognize physical changes of aging
- ☐ Identify reactions to death and dying

| Part 1 | # Confusion |

A confused patient feels insecure and frustrated.

Confusion is not a disease; it is a side effect of other problems. Confusion is caused by a decreased blood supply to the brain or loss of brain cells which can result from severe emotional stress, disease, infection, medication, or injury. It is important to chart the first time a patient shows confused behavior; it may be a warning sign of stroke, dehydration, or fever.

The confused patient may need to be reminded of daily activities such as eating, bathing, dressing, and toileting. The patient may become fearful and frustrated.

Reality orientation is a major part of caring for the confused patient. Repetition is very important.

- Repeat the person's name often.
- Identify yourself each time you visit the patient.
- Always speak slowly and calmly.
- Use simple words that the patient understands.
- Repeat the day, date, and time often.
- Put calendars and clocks where the patient can see them easily.
- Open the drapes during the day and close them at night.
- Discuss familiar people, objects, and events.

- Encourage the patient to watch TV and listen to the radio.
- Protect the patient from injury; he or she may not be aware of hazards.
- Give instructions that are easy to follow, and repeat as often as necessary.
- Ask simple questions and allow time for the response.
- Never rush the patient.
- Maintain a predictable routine and be consistent.
- Avoid changing furniture, and keep familiar pictures visible.
- Provide quiet.
- Watch the patient closely to prevent wandering.

Mental retardation is caused by brain damage. Mentally retarded patients may be confused, and they are limited in what they can learn. Mildly retarded patients can learn self-care with assistance. Severely retarded patients are dependent on others for their care.

Treat patients who are mentally retarded the same as other patients, and encourage them to participate in social activities. If the patient is confused, use reality orientation.

| Part 2 | # Alzheimer's Disease |

Alzheimer's is a disease that affects normal functioning of the brain.

The cause of **Alzheimer's disease** (AD) is unknown, and there is no cure. The disease affects the part of the brain related to memory, thinking, and judgment. Communication is disrupted as **dementia** (loss of mental ability) gets steadily worse. Use reality orientation with AD patients.

Phases of Alzheimer's Disease

AD is a terminal illness that affects each patient differently. In general, the disease becomes increasingly worse in three phases.

Phase one may not be immediately noticeable. The patient has less energy and less enthusiasm for life. Reactions are slow, judgment is impaired, and decisions may be difficult. The patient forgets recent events.

In **phase two** the patient functions; however, math calculations (balancing a checkbook or paying bills) are very difficult. The patient becomes disoriented — unable to remember people and places — and experiences difficulty in speaking and understanding. Restlessness is common, with an increasingly shorter attention span and loss of memory.

In **phase three** the patient cannot perform the activities of daily living (such as bathing, toileting, dressing). Directions need to be repeated and still may not be understood. The patient may have outbursts of anger or tears. Extreme confusion may be present. The patient loses the ability to speak and cannot recognize family members. Body functions decline and the patient is dependent upon care until death.

Part 3   # Cancer

Side effects of cancer treatment impact
a patient physically and emotionally.

Cancer is a **malignant tumor**, a growth that spreads and destroys. Treatment is aimed at destroying the tumor.

Some cancers are treated with **radiation therapy** (high-energy rays) or **chemotherapy** (drugs) over a prolonged period of time.

Caring for the Cancer Patient

Provide both physical and emotional support. Take time to listen if the patient wants to talk. Show compassion and understanding, and be alert to the side effects of cancer treatment. Encourage activities (such as knitting and crafts).

Nutrition

Treatment can cause nausea and vomiting, and the patient may lose all interest in food.

- Provide nutritious foods even if the patient is not hungry.
- Encourage the patient to eat frequent small meals.
- Encourage the patient to take small amounts of highly nutritional liquid supplements that may be ordered.
- Notify the supervisor if severe nausea and vomiting persist.

Dry Mouth

Soothe a dry mouth by offering the patient fluids and soft foods.

- Offer cooling foods (ice cream, melon, popsicles, apple juice) if allowed.
- Avoid citrus juices that may cause irritation.
- Serve soft food, or cut food into small pieces.
- Provide hard candy to moisten the mouth.
- Help keep the patient's mouth clean.

Fatigue

It is normal for the patient to tire easily.

- Encourage plenty of rest, but do not ignore the patient.
- Let the patient know it is normal to tire easily.
- Offer understanding and support.

Hair Loss

Hair loss is common and has a strong emotional impact.

- Encourage the patient to wear a pretty scarf or wig.
- Accept the patient's temporary baldness, and try to ease feelings of self-consciousness.

Skin Sensitivity

The skin becomes easily irritated. Rashes and sores are common.

- Help the patient to reposition often.
- Avoid coarse blankets that may rub the skin.
- Do not use talcum powder; it contains metals that irritate.

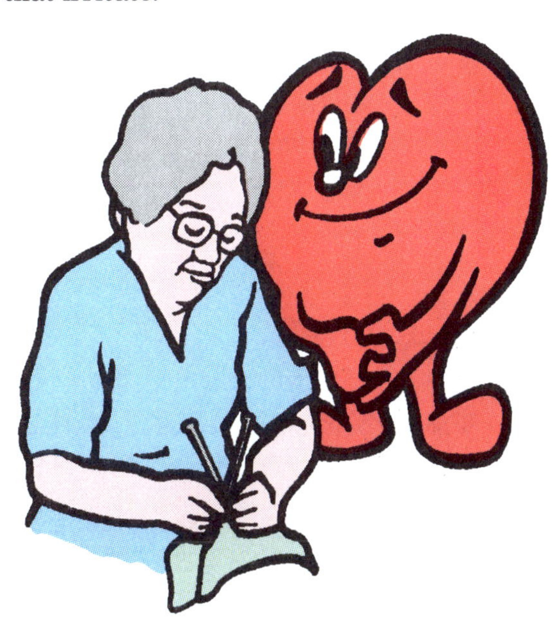

<table><tr><td>Part 4</td><td><h1>Diabetes</h1></td></tr></table>

Diabetes can be controlled through diet, exercise, and medication.

Diabetes results when the body cannot produce enough **insulin**. Insulin is a hormone produced by the pancreas to help the body break down and convert sugars and starches into energy.

Symptoms of Diabetes

- thirst
- frequent urination
- fatigue
- skin is easily irritated and slow to heal
- blurred vision
- weight loss
- muscle cramps

Caring for the Diabetic Patient

- Monitor the patient's food intake and report any food not consumed.
- Protect against cuts and scrapes. Diabetics heal slowly and are susceptible to infection. Severe infections could result in amputation.
- Report any complaints of pain immediately.
- Report any change in activity or food intake. Insulin dosages may need to be altered to compensate for changes.
- Be sure clothing and bed coverings do not cut off blood circulation.
- Provide good skin care.
- Report any changes in skin color or temperature.

Complications

Hyperglycemia (diabetic coma) is the result of too little insulin or too much sugar. It occurs when blood sugar levels are high and **acidosis** (inability of the body to excrete toxins) is present. Though the onset is gradual, this is a life-threatening condition requiring immediate care.

Early Signs of Hyperglycemia

- increased urination
- abdominal pain
- thirst
- nausea
- drowsiness

Later Signs

- heavy breathing
- flushed face
- breath has a fruity scent
- dry skin
- loss of consciousness
- death

Treatment

- Insulin is injected by a licensed nurse.
- Stay with the person and offer support.
- Report any abnormal symptoms immediately.

Hypoglycemia (insulin shock) is a condition resulting from too much insulin or too little sugar. There is danger of insulin shock when too much insulin has been taken or too little food is consumed. Hypoglycemia comes on very quickly.

Signs of Hypoglycemia

- hunger
- lethargy, weakness, dizziness
- sweating
- trembling
- unconsciousness
- death

Treatment

Glucose (sugar) is given orally. In severe cases, glucose may be injected **intravenously** (into the vein) by a licensed nurse.

<table><tr><td>Part 5</td><td></td></tr></table>

Heart Disease

*Heart disease is caused by a breakdown
in the body's pumping system.*

The cardiovascular system is the pumping system of the body. The heart is the pump; and the veins, arteries, and **capillaries** (blood vessels) carry blood, oxygen, and nutrients throughout the system.

Causes of Heart Problems

Heart disease occurs when the heart no longer pumps efficiently or the blood supply to vital organs is reduced due to blockage of blood vessels.

Arteriosclerosis (hardening of the arteries) occurs when the arteries thicken with age.

Atherosclerosis (blockage) is when arteries become clogged with deposits such as *cholesterol, calcium,* or *fat.*

Both conditions prevent sufficient blood from reaching the heart, brain, and other vital organs. When the blood supply to the heart is reduced, parts of the heart muscle die, causing **myocardial infarction (MI)**, known as a heart attack.

Signs of a Heart Attack

If a patient complains of any of these symptoms, report it immediately!

- pain in the chest
- numbness or pain in the left arm and neck
- irregular pulse rate (weak or fast)
- decrease in blood pressure
- difficulty in breathing
- dizziness
- pale, clammy skin

Caring for the Heart Patient

Make the patient comfortable.

- Position the patient in bed to make breathing easier.
- Raise the head and chest.
- Place pillows to support the arms and neck.
- If the patient must be moved, be gentle.

Allow the patient to rest.

- Avoid unnecessary activity.
- Anticipate the patient's needs.
- Keep the room pleasant and quiet.

Ensure the proper use of oxygen.

- Check the tank balance often.
- Know all safety precautions in handling oxygen.
- If the patient has difficulty breathing, report it immediately.

Observe proper diet guidelines.

- Be sure the prescribed diet is followed.

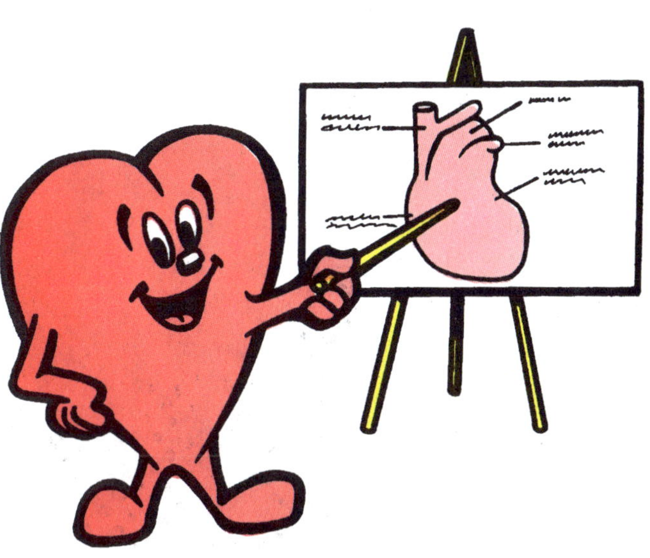

Pacemakers

A healthy heart regulates heart beats with a **pacemaker**, a specialized mass of muscle fibers. A heart that does not function properly may require an artificial pacemaker to be placed surgically in the person's chest.

Artificial Pacemakers

The **demand** pacemaker is used when the patient has a history of irregular heart rate. The heart is stimulated only when the rate drops below a preset level.

The **fixed-rate** pacemaker is used when the heart is completely dependent on artificial stimulation. The rate is usually set at 60-70 beats per minute.

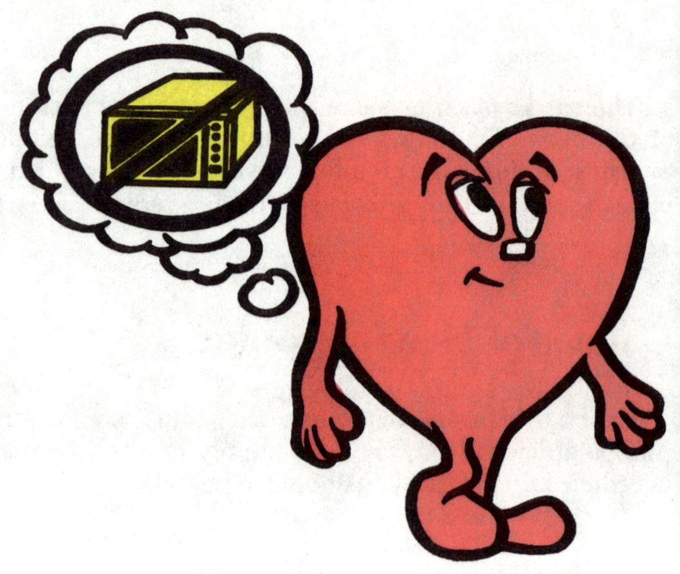

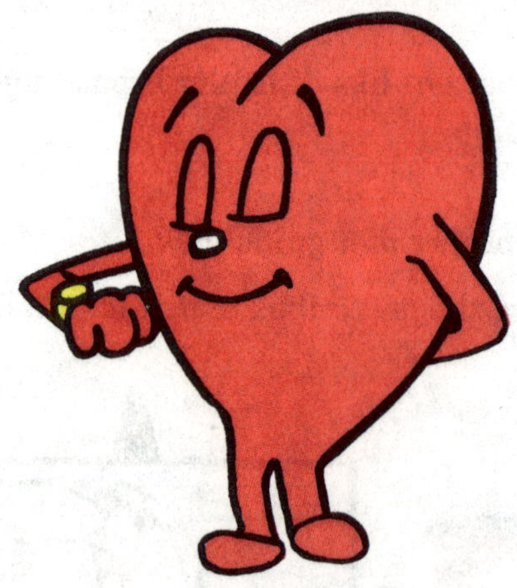

Caring for the Patient with an Artificial Pacemaker

- Know the patient's set heart rate. If the rate falls below the set rate, report it to your supervisor immediately.

- Check for edema, pain, or dizziness.

- Look for discoloration in the area of the pacemaker.

- Report hiccups immediately. Hiccups may indicate that the pacemaker is out of place.

- Do not use microwave ovens near people with pacemakers.

- Electrical appliances (razors, televisions) should be used with caution.

Part 6 — Seizures

Patients need your help to protect them from injury during seizures.

A **seizure** (sudden attack) results when normal brain cell activity is disrupted. Seizures can happen to anyone.

Seizures may be caused by:

- tumors
- head injury
- fever
- chemical imbalance
- stroke

When no specific reason can be found for a seizure, the condition is called **epilepsy**. Epilepsy is not contagious, nor does it affect the mind. People with epilepsy may have grand mal or petit mal seizures, or epilepsy may be completely controlled with medication.

Types of Seizures

Grand mal seizures involve the whole body with **convulsions** (jerking of muscles) and loss of consciousness. Seizures may last for several minutes.

Petit mal is a partial seizure. The patient does not lose consciousness and may appear to be day dreaming. There may be some shaking or jerking of muscles. Seizures last only a few seconds and occur frequently.

Psychomotor includes temporary loss of judgment and muscular control.

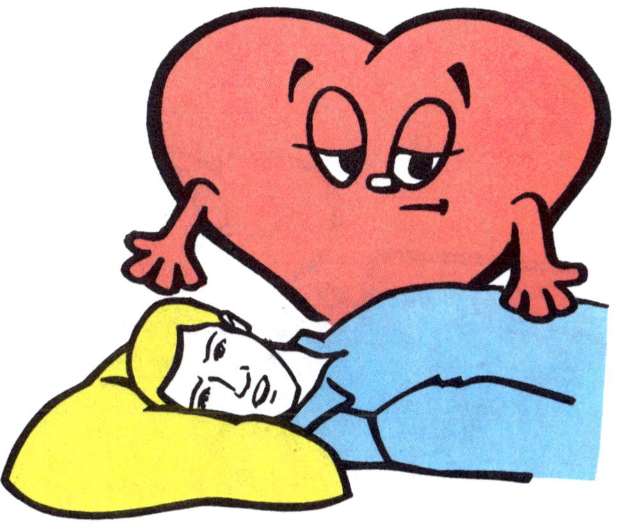

Caring for the Patient During a Seizure

1. Call for help.

2. Do whatever is necessary to protect the patient from injury.

3. Do not leave the patient.

4. Help the patient lie down.

5. Place a pillow under the head.

6. If possible, turn the head to one side to prevent choking.

7. Move furniture and equipment out of the way if the seizure occurs on the floor.

8. If the patient is in bed, pad the side rails with blankets or soft foam.

Do not try to restrain the patient.
Do not pry the mouth open.
Do not insert anything into the mouth.

Caring for the Patient After a Seizure

1. Be aware that the patient will not remember the seizure.

2. Help the patient into bed.

3. Put up the side rails for protection.

4. Offer comfort and support.

5. Report all seizures to your supervisor.

6. Chart that the seizure was observed and reported.

<table>
<tr><td>Part 7</td><td><h1 align="center">Stroke</h1></td></tr>
</table>

Aging increases the chance of cerebral vascular accident (CVA), also known as stroke.

Cerebral (brain) **vascular** (blood vessels) accident, called CVA or stroke, results from a variety of physical problems:

Blockage	blocks the blood vessels, reducing the blood supply to the brain
Thrombus	a blood clot in the brain
Embolus	a blood clot carried to the brain through the circulatory system
Rupture	bleeding in the brain

Effects of a Stroke

Many stroke patients lose control of muscles and thought processes. They may know what they want but not be able to say or write the words. A stroke victim may say "yes" and mean "no."

Hemiplegia (paralysis on one side) is common after a stroke. Paralysis occurs on the side of the body opposite the affected part of the brain. In other words, a stroke on the right side of the brain affects the left side of the body.

Hemiparesis is a loss of sensation in the affected side. The patient is able to move, but has no feeling in the limbs. Danger of burns, scrapes, and other injuries are present with hemiparesis.

Other symptoms of a stroke:

• eyelid and mouth may droop

• arm bends across chest

• wrist bends with fingers curled inward

• **spasms** (involuntary muscle contractions) may occur in the paralyzed limbs

Stages of Recovery

There are three progressive stages in the treatment of stroke victims. Not all patients experience each stage.

Flaccid	the affected side remains limp and weak
Spastic	the affected side develops some tense muscles, with frequent spasms
Recovery	the affected side regains normal use

Caring for the Stroke Patient

1. Encourage as much independence as possible.

2. Encourage the patient to exercise joints to prevent **atrophy** (wasting away of muscles).

3. Help reposition the patient often to prevent bedsores.

4. Prevent injury by providing safety measures (bed rails, walkers).

5. Provide good skin care.

6. Give good mouth care.

7. Be patient and supportive.

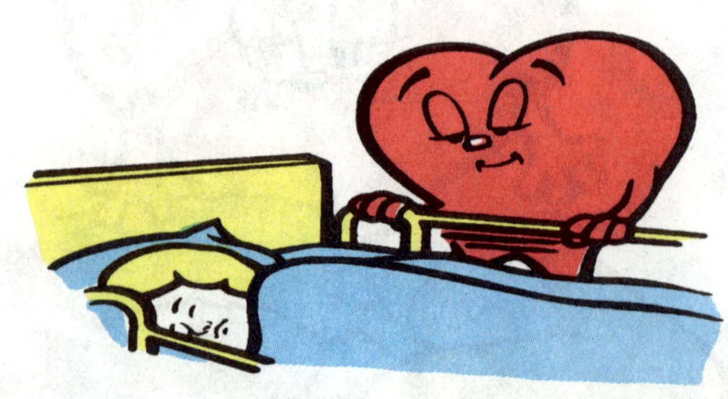

Part 8 — Physical Changes Related to Aging

Help patients adapt to the physical changes of aging.

System	What Happens	What to Do
Cardiovascular	• heart muscle loses strength • arteries/veins get narrower, reduce blood flow • less oxygen to entire body • slower healing	Work with the health-care team to develop an exercise program. Encourage exercise based on the patient's care plan. Report tiring from exercises.
Nervous	• loss of brain cells • less blood to brain • forgets recent events • confusion, dizziness	Don't rush the patient. Allow time for decisions. Avoid abrupt schedule changes. Encourage thinking, reading, mental exercises.
Sensory	• reduced vision, hearing • decreased taste, smell • reduced sense of touch, less likely to feel pain • voice muscles lose strength	Encourage use of glasses and hearing aids if needed. Speak slowly and clearly. Listen carefully when the patient speaks. Encourage good nutrition even though the food may not taste good to the patient.
Respiratory	• lungs lose strength • more lung deposits possible • harder to breathe	Get patient out of bed often. Encourage exercise. Use light bed covers. Occasional coughing clears lungs.
Musculoskeletal	• muscles atrophy, lose strength • bones lose density, get more brittle • joints less flexible • gradual height loss	Avoid falls; hip fractures can be deadly. Position and walk as indicated in the patient's care plan.
Skin/ Integumentary	• skin drys, less elastic • wrinkles, age spots appear • skin loses fatty layer so person gets cooler • surface blood vessels weaken • nails thicken, toughen • hair turns gray, falls out • skin bruises easily	If bedridden, change positions frequently to help prevent bedsores. Smooth wrinkles from linens. Keep skin clean and dry. Use lotions for moisture. Remove safety hazards to prevent skin damage. Use extreme care clipping nails. Layer bed covers for warmth.
Digestive	• less saliva production • more difficulty swallowing • loss of teeth, harder to chew • less taste, less appetite • more frequent constipation • more indigestion	Encourage fluids. Allow plenty of time to eat. Make sure dentures are in place if used. Encourage frequent toileting and establish bowel movement regularity.
Urinary	• reduced kidney function • less bladder control, incontinence • more frequent urination	Encourage daytime drinking of fluids. If the patient is incontinent, do not criticize. Follow bladder training program.
Reproductive	• less ability to get, maintain erection in men • menopause in women • reduced vaginal lubrication	Recognize that people of all ages are sexual beings. Allow time and privacy for a patient's sex life. Be willing to discuss sex openly. Never tease, criticize, or embarrass a patient.
Endocrine	• decreased hormone levels • less body water so weight loss • less ability to handle stress • more likely to become ill • takes longer to get well	Wash hands often and well. Keep surroundings clean to prevent infection. Reduce stress and schedule changes. Offer encouragement, not criticism.

Part 9 — Dealing with Death and Dying

Fear is a common reaction to death.

As an NA, you will care for patients in the last stages of life. Do not allow your fear of death to stop you from being sensitive to the patient's needs. Offer concerned care and understanding.

If you have lost a loved one, think about how you felt. Consider how death was handled by the family, medical staff, and friends. Reflect on what comforted you and what upset you. Use your experiences to help your patients.

- Make the patient as comfortable as possible.
- Continue normal care.
- Do not leave the patient alone.
- Keep the room well lighted; darkness may be frightening.
- Keep the room well ventilated.
- Talk in a normal voice.
- Do not tiptoe.
- Provide comfort and support for the patient and the family.
- Respect the need for time and privacy with close family and friends.
- Provide spiritual support if requested (according to the facility's procedures).
- Allow the patient to die with dignity.

Stages of Grief

Patients who believe they are about to die react in different ways. Moods may change from day to day as they grieve over life ending. Family members may experience the same feelings.

In her work with dying patients, Dr. Elizabeth Kubler-Ross identified five stages of grief. The stages apply to any major loss.

- denial
- depression
- anger
- bargaining
- acceptance

Not everyone goes through all five stages, nor is there a specific order. Some may repeat stages. Being familiar with the five stages of grief will help you understand what the patient and family are experiencing.

Denial is a state of shock when the patient cannot accept what is happening. The patient may insist it is a mistake or may ignore the facts completely.

- Do not force people to face the truth.
- Give people time to adjust.
- Listen when people want to talk.
- Do not force conversation.

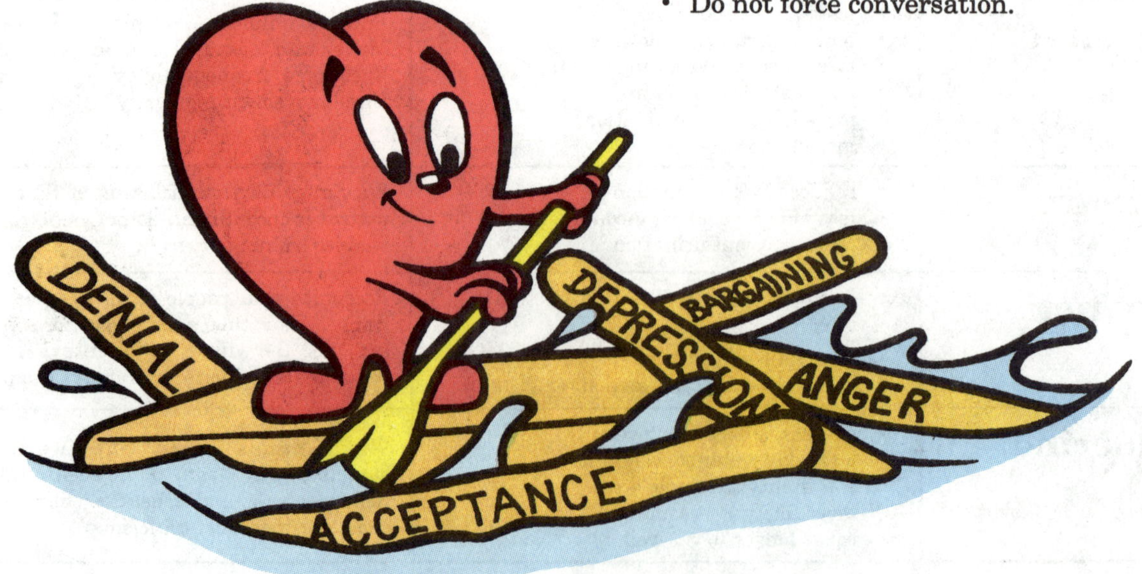

Anger is normal. People express anger at God, at the doctor, at life, perhaps even at you. Patients may yell at you, accuse you of poor care, complain about everything, or refuse to do anything you ask.

- Be patient.
- Continue giving the best care you can.
- Do not take insults personally.
- Do not become defensive.

Depression happens when people have partially accepted death. They are sorting out their feelings. Sometimes people become very withdrawn, and may not want to eat or socialize. Others become more talkative and need more of your time.

- Being there for the patient is very important. If he or she wants to talk, listen patiently.
- Be compassionate. If the patient does not want to talk, do not force conversation.
- Give the best nursing care you can.

Bargaining is when people try to make deals to postpone death. They will bargain with God or the doctors. Sometimes they may try to bargain with you.

- Listen with a caring attitude.
- Never make promises or say, "Things will be all right."
- Let the patients know you are there for them.
- Hold the patient's hand for comfort.

Acceptance is when the patient accepts that death is inevitable. It does not mean that he or she wants to die. The patient may be talkative or very quiet. Spending time with close relatives or friends may be very comforting for the patient.

- Just being there to hold a hand and keep the patient from feeling alone is a comfort.
- Continue routine care.
- Provide privacy with loved ones.
- If a clergy member is requested, let your supervisor know immediately.

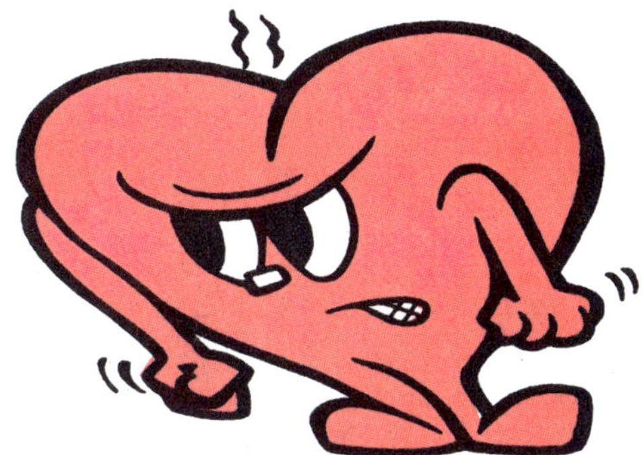

Care of the Body After Death

Postmortem (after death) care begins as soon as the patient is pronounced dead. A licensed **nurse is** usually responsible for postmortem care. The NA may be asked to assist. The right to be treated with respect and dignity and the right to privacy apply after death as well as during life.

- Position the body in normal alignment.
- Close the eyes gently.
- Insert dentures if appropriate.
- Close the mouth.
- Cover the body to the shoulders with a sheet if the family is to view the body.

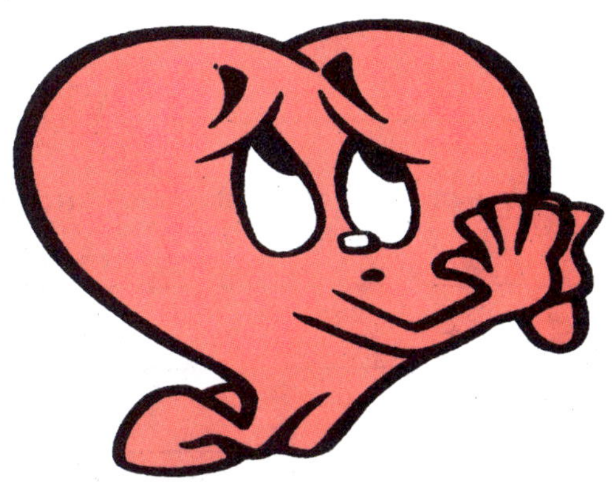

NA Review

1. How can the NA help the patient who is suffering from confusion?

____

____

____

____

2. Identify the three phases of Alzheimer's Disease.

____

____

____

3. Discuss some ways to help the cancer patient cope with the side-effects of treatment.

____

____

____

____

4. Identify symptoms of diabetes.

____

____

____

____

5. Identify three or more signs of a heart attack.

1) Pain in left arm and neck.

____

____

6. How would you prevent injury to the patient during a seizure?

____

____

____

____

7. Identify the stages of recovery for a stroke victim.

____

____

____

____

8. Discuss physical changes related to aging.

____

____

____

____

9. Describe the stages of grief.

____

____

____

____

Vocabulary

acidosis	(as-i-**do**-sis)	inability of blood to get rid of toxins
artery	(**ar**-ter-ee)	blood vessel that carries blood away from heart
atherosclerosis	(ath-ur-o-skle-**ro**-sis)	blockage of the arteries
capillaries	(**kap**-i-lair-eez)	tiny blood vessels
cerebral vascular accident	(**ser**-e-brul **vas**-ku-lar)	stroke
chemotherapy	(kem-o-**ther**-ah-pee)	treatment using drugs
dementia	(de-**men**-she-ah)	mental abilities steadily worsen
diabetes	(dy-ah-**be**-teez)	too much or too little sugar in blood
embolus	(**em**-bo-lus)	blood clot carried to brain
epilepsy	(**ep**-i-lep-see)	chronic disease with seizures
flaccid	(**flak**-sid)	weak and limp
hemiparesis	(hem-i-**par**-e-sis)	loss of sensation in one side of body after stroke
hypoglycemia	(hy-po-gly-**see**-me-ah)	too much insulin or too little sugar
hyperglycemia	(hy-per-gly-**see**-me-ah)	too little insulin or too much sugar
integumentary	(in-teg-yoo-**men**-ter-ee)	skin
insulin	(**in**-su-lin)	hormone produced by pancreas to break down sugars and starches
myocardial infarction	(my-o-**kar**-dee-ul in-**fark**-shun)	heart attack
psychomotor	(sy-ko-**mo**-tor)	temporary loss of judgment and muscle control
radiation	(ray-dee-**ay**-shun)	treatment using high-energy waves
thrombus	(**throm**-bus)	blood clot in the brain

Additional Terms to Remember

____

____

NA Notes

Reality orientation is for patients who have lost their short-term memory and cannot recall recent events.

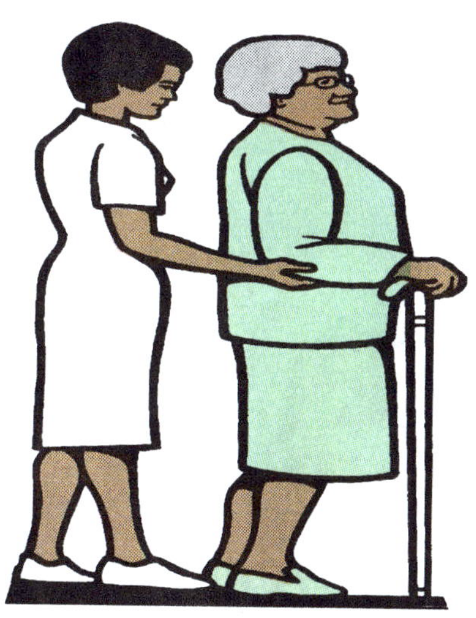

Assistive Devices

Help your patients keep their independence!

Objectives:

- ☐ Demonstrate proper care for assistive devices
- ☐ Describe preventive care and maintenance for hearing aids
- ☐ Discuss ways to help patients keep track of glasses
- ☐ Identify mobility aids
- ☐ Recognize the proper use of canes
- ☐ Explain the proper use of walkers

Part 1   **Proper Care for Assistive Devices**

Assistive devices help the patients rely more on themselves and less on the NA.

Assistive devices such as glasses, hearing aids, walkers, canes, and wheelchairs contribute to a patient's well-being and independence. A **prosthesis** is an artificial body part such as an arm, leg, breast, or eye. Proper care and use of assistive devices and prostheses is important.

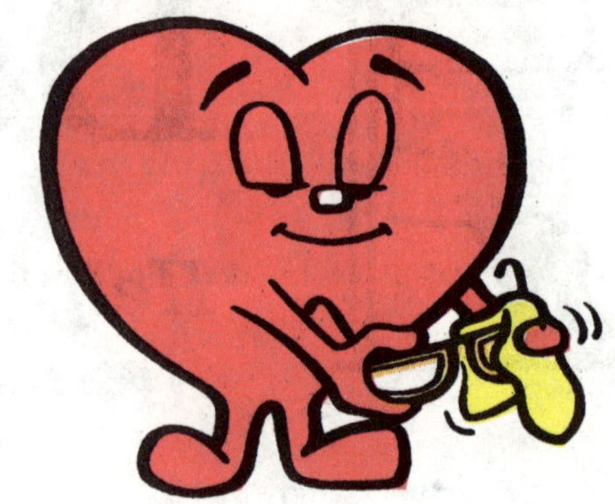

- Know proper handling of a device before helping a patient.

- Make sure the patient knows how to use the device.

- Inspect the device before and after use, making sure it is in good condition. DO NOT let a patient use a defective device.

- Keep the patient's equipment within easy reach.

- Check for any physical problems that might develop with use (pinching, swelling, rubbing, sore spots).

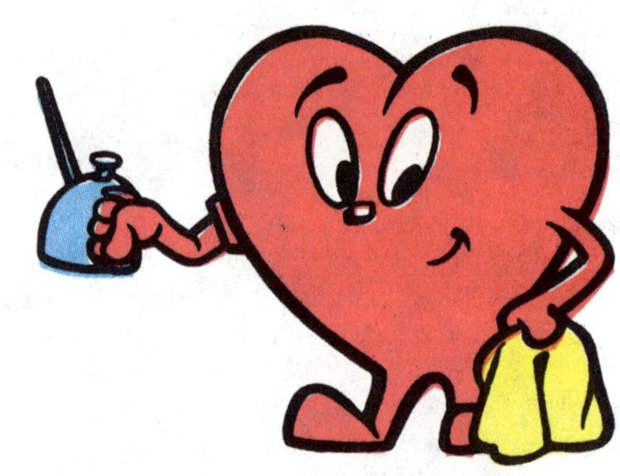

- Keep the device properly cleaned.

- Schedule regular maintenance.

- Mark the patient's name in an inconspicuous place for identification.

- Mark the removeable foot pedals on wheelchairs.

- Encourage patients to help with the care of devices if they are able.

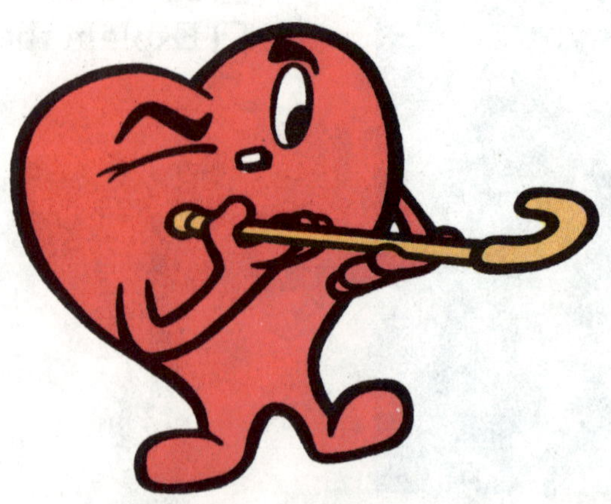

<table><tr><td>Part 2</td><td></td></tr></table>

Hearing Aids

Hearing aids are fragile and require special care.

Be cautious when you handle hearing aids. For example, use a table or desk for cleaning or changing batteries. Dropping a hearing aid causes damage.

Keep hearing aids dry; water ruins them.

- Remove hearing aids before showering or swimming.
- If the aid gets wet, dry it with a soft cloth; never use heat.

Keep hearing aids clean.

- Use a soft cloth.
- Never use oil.
- Never use water, alcohol, or cleaning solvents.
- Remove the aid before using hair spray.

Extend the life of batteries; they are expensive.

- Turn off the hearing aid when it is not in use.
- Open the door to disconnect the battery contact for nighttime storage.
- Remove the battery if the aid will not be used for over 24 hours.
- Check to be sure the battery is working before placing the aid in a patient's ear.

Store hearing aids in a safe place.

- Always use a case for storing the hearing aid.
- Mark the case with the patient's name.
- Never leave it within reach of visiting children.
- Discourage the patient from putting it in a pocket; it may go to the laundry with the clothing!

Hearing Aid Trouble Shooting

Problem	Possible Cause	Action
Doesn't Work	dead battery plugged earmold	replace battery clean earmold
Not Loud Enough	low battery plugged earmold hearing may have changed	replace battery clean earmold have hearing checked
Distorted	low battery	replace battery
Fuzzy	faulty hearing aid	check with dispenser
Goes On and Off	bad battery faulty hearing aid	replace battery check with dispenser
Causes Discomfort	improperly placed wrong style	check placement check with dispenser

<table><tr><td>Part 3</td><td># Vision Aids</td></tr></table>

Protect the patient's possessions from damage or loss.

Glasses

Glasses are often misplaced or broken.

- Engrave the patient's name on the inside of the frame.

- Make sure the patient has a case on the nightstand for storing glasses. A second case may be needed to carry glasses during the day.

- Provide a neckstrap to keep glasses within easy reach for those who frequently take glasses on and off.

- Avoid scratches by cleaning glasses with a soft cloth. Paper tissues scratch lenses.

- Check glasses often for loose screws or broken nosepieces.

Artificial Eyes

Artificial eyes are cared for by the nursing staff unless the patient's flow sheet states otherwise. If the NA cleans an artificial eye, it must be handled carefully to prevent scratching or breaking. Wash your hands before handling the eye.

- Clean the eye over a sink or basin half filled with warm water to avoid breakage if dropped.

- Wet the eye under warm running water.

- Rub the eye *gently* with clean sterile gauze.

- Rinse the eye under the running water.

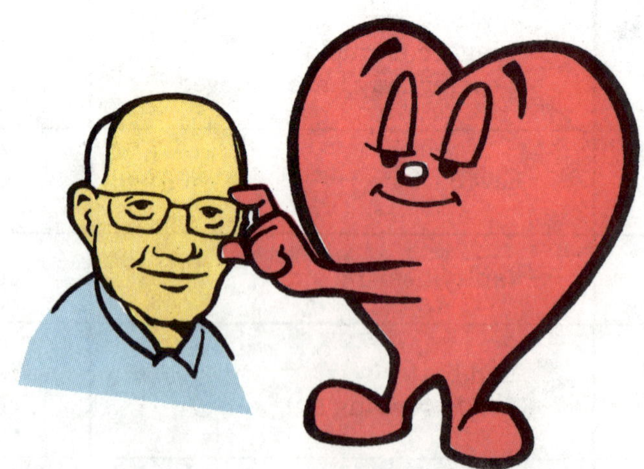

<table><tr><td>Part 4</td><td># Devices to Aid Mobility</td></tr></table>

Mobility devices increase the patient's independence.

Many patients use assistive devices for mobility. The NA is responsible for observing and reporting any problems in using the equipment and any repairs that are needed.

Wheelchairs

When using a wheelchair, be sure the patient is properly positioned for comfort and safety.

Wheelchairs are equipped with a variety of options:

- removable arm rests
- heel loops to prevent feet from slipping off
- special seat cushions

Proper Care for Wheelchairs

- Check for loose, worn, or missing parts.
- Check the brakes.
- Oil metal parts once a week.
- Keep the chair clean.
- Be sure the chair is properly adjusted for the patient.

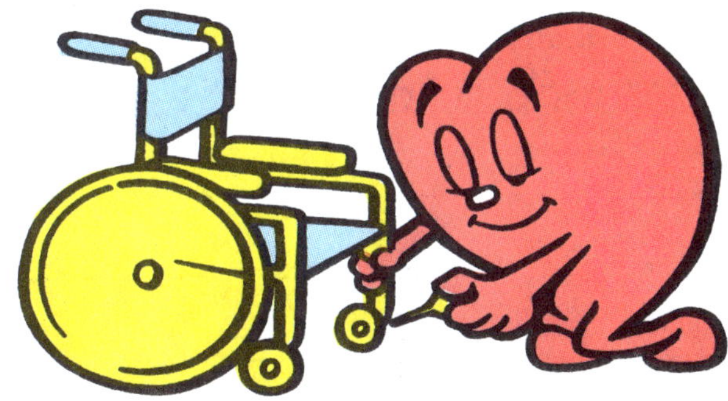

Canes

Canes are used for balance or to support weight.

- For balance, the cane is carried on the patient's strong side.
- For supporting weight, the cane is carried on the weak side.

Proper care for canes:

- Check the tips for worn cups.
- Check canes for cracks or loose screws.
- Be sure the patient is using the cane properly.

Walkers

The type of walker that is used depends on the patient's individual needs and ability. Walkers are ordered by a doctor or physical therapist.

The **standard walker** is rigid with four legs. It is used for balance and has suction-cup safety tips.

The **gliding walker** is the same as the **standard** walker except there are wheels on the front legs. The walker can be pushed without having to pick it up.

Caution: the wheels may roll out from under the patient, causing a fall.

The **reciprocal walker** has a hinged frame and moves forward one side at a time. It has suction-cup safety tips.

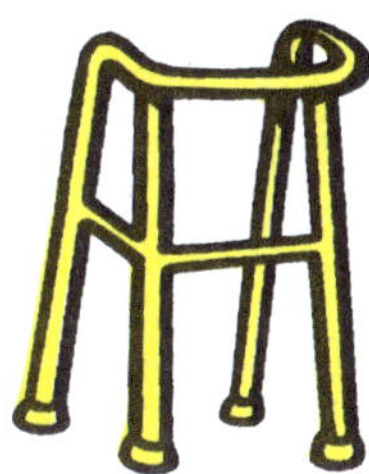

Proper Care for Walkers

- Make sure the walker is the correct size for the patient.
- Check for loose screws.
- Check for worn suction cups or tips.

Crutches

Occasionally patients use crutches. Patients who use crutches should be checked regularly for friction sores.

Proper Care for Crutches

- Check the crutch tips.
- Check the padding for wear.
- Check for loose screws or cracks.

NA Review

1. Describe how to care for assistive devices.

2. Describe proper maintenance for hearing aids.

3. Identify ways to prevent losing glasses.

4. What are three or more safety precautions for wheelchairs?

   1) Check the brakes.

5. What are some safety precautions for canes and walkers?

Vocabulary

| artificial | (ar-ti-**fish**-ul) | a copy or substitute |
| prosthesis | (pros-**thee**-sis) | artificial body part |

Additional Terms to Remember

NA Notes

Never allow a patient to use a defective devise.

Practical Skills for the NA

Your training includes hands-on performance and practice.

To pass the certification exam, the NA must be able to demonstrate skills for providing quality services to patients.

Go through the following list and check off those skills you feel confident you can perform to the best of your ability. Work on those you leave unchecked.

- ☐ Maintains and respects patient rights regardless of race, religion, or life-style.
- ☐ Promotes self-care and independence based on the patient's capabilities.
- ☐ Recognizes the patient's right to decisions about personal care.
- ☐ Respects the patient's need for privacy and confidentiality.
- ☐ Reports the patient's concerns.
- ☐ Demonstrates safety and emergency procedures.
- ☐ Identifies common basic needs.
- ☐ Assists the patient in getting to and participating in activities.
- ☐ Demonstrates communication and interpersonal skills.
- ☐ Accurately records and promptly reports pertinent observations, using appropriate terms.
- ☐ Explains how disease-causing microorganisms are spread.
- ☐ Demonstrates procedures for infection control (including handwashing).
- ☐ Provides care and security for the patient's personal possessions.
- ☐ Measures and records vital signs.
- ☐ Measures and records height and weight.
- ☐ Measures and records fluid and food intake and output.
- ☐ Evaluates food and fluid needs.
- ☐ Recognizes and reports abnormal signs and symptoms.
- ☐ Uses correct charting procedures.
- ☐ Shows sensitivity to emotional, social, and mental health needs.
- ☐ Demonstrates good judgment in emergencies.

☐ Demonstrates basic patient care:
    bed making
    bathing
    perineal care
    mouth care
    skin care
    nail care
    grooming
    dressing
    toileting
    feeding and hydrating
    elimination
    range of motion
    lifting, turning, positioning, and transferring

☐ Uses good body mechanics for self and patients.

☐ Provides a clean, orderly, and safe environment for the patients.

☐ Demonstrates the proper use and storage of cleaning and hazardous materials.

☐ Provides adequate ventilation, warmth, light, and quiet.

☐ Demonstrates proper care and use of assistive devices (hearing aids, glasses, ambulation, artificial limbs, eating utensils, dressing aids).

☐ Identifies developmental tasks of aging and adjusts for physical and mental limitations.

☐ Displays mature response with issues involving sexuality.

☐ Recognizes how family and friends influence the patient's behavior and care.

☐ Provides care and behavior that minimize the need for physical or chemical restraints.

☐ Makes sure that the patient is free from abuse, mistreatment, or neglect, and reports instances to appropriate staff.

☐ Accepts responsibility for own actions, and recognizes the affect of own behavior on the patient's behavior.

☐ Recognizes behavior related to the grieving process.

☐ Demonstrates appropriate care for the dying patient.

☐ Works within the NA job description.

☐ Demonstrates the ability to work cooperatively with the health-care team and to follow instructions.

Medical Abbreviations

Knowing medical abbreviations helps save time when filling out and reading patient charts.

ā	before	ENT	ears, nose, throat
abd	abdomen	FF	force fluids
a.c.	before meals	ft	feet
AD	Alzheimer's Disease	Fx	fracture
ADL	activities of daily living	G.I.	gastrointestinal
ad lib	as desired	G.U.	genitourinary
a.m.	morning	H_2O	water
amb	ambulate	h.s.	bedtime (hour of sleep)
amt	amount	HOH	hard of hearing
ax	axillary (armpit)	ht	height
b.i.d.	two times a day	in	inch
BM	bowel movement	I/O	intake and output
BP	blood pressure	IV	intravenous
BRP	bathroom privileges	L	liter
c̄	with	lb	pound
Ca	cancer	lt	left
cc	cubic centimeter	LPN	licensed practical nurse
CBR	complete bed rest	MI	myocardial infarction
CHF	congestive heart failure	mm	millimeters
CN	charge nurse	noc	night
c/o	complains of	NPO	nothing by mouth
CVA	cerebral vascular accident (stroke)	O_2	oxygen
DC	discontinue	oz	ounce
DON	director of nursing	p̄	after
Dr.	doctor	pc	after meals
Dx	diagnosis	po	by mouth (oral)
EEG	electroencephalogram	p.m.	afternoon or evening
EKG or ECG	electrocardiogram	p.r.n.	as necessary

pt	patient		SOB	shortness of breath
PT	physical therapy		staph	staphylococcus (germ)
q.d.	every day		STAT	immediately
q.i.d.	four times a day		tab	tablet
q.h.	every hour		tbsp	tablespoon
q.o.d.	every other day		t.i.d.	three times a day
R	rectal		TPR	temperature, pulse, respiration
RBC	red blood count		tsp	teaspoon
RN	registered nurse		U/A	urinalysis
ROM	range of motion		URI	upper respiratory infection
rt	right		UTI	urinary tract infection
Rx	prescription		V.S.	vital signs
$\bar{s}$	without		WBC	white blood count
S/A	suger/acetone (urine test)		W/C	wheelchair
spec	specimen		wt	weight

Practical Use of Abbreviations

Examples

1. amb $\bar{c}$ walker b.i.d.
   ambulate with walker two times a day

2. dresses $\bar{s}$ supervision
   dresses without supervision

3. elevate head of bed p.r.n. SOB
   raise head of bed as needed for shortness of breath

4. assist $\bar{c}$ ROM exercise t.i.d.
   assist with range-of-motion exercises three times a day

5. give 1 tab t.i.d. ac
   give one tablet three times a day before meals

Practice

1. Pt c/o headache

   ____

2. Report to CN STAT

   ____

3. TPR b.i.d.

   ____

4. Amb q.i.d.

   ____

5. Reposition pt q.h.

   ____

Bibliographical Resources

American Red Cross, *American Red Cross Nurse Assistant Training*, 1989.

Anderson, Samuel L., M.D., *The New Home Medical Encyclopedia*, Volume 2, Quadrangle Books, 1973.

Back Tips for Health Care Providers, Krames Communications, California, 1986.

Berg, Karin, Patti Kratzke, Edna Olufson, Peggy Mouser and Kitty Peck, *City University Nursing Assistant Certification*, City University Press, Seattle, Washington,1982.

Consumer Guide, *Family Medical & Health Guide*, Publications Int'l., Lincolnwood, Illinois, 1985.

Daniels, Leola, *Competencies for Nursing Assistants - A Curriculum Guide*, Idaho, 1989.

Gillogly, Barbara, *Skills and Techniques for the New Nursing Assistant*, Medcom, Inc. and Quality Care Health Foundation, California, 1990.

Good Housekeeping, *The New Good Housekeeping Health and Medical Guide*, Hearst Corporation, New York, 1989.

Kubler-Ross, Elizabeth, *On Death and Dying*, Macmillan, New York, 1969.

Mace, Nancy and Peter Rabins, *The 36 Hour Day*, Johns Hopkins University, Baltimore, Maryland, 1983.

Maslow, Abraham, *Toward a Psychology of Being*, 2nd Ed., D. Van Nostrand, Princeton, New Jersey, 1962.

Mullen, Lynn and Janet Fouts, *Nursing Assistant Training Manual*, Oregon Medical Express, Beaverton, Oregon, 1989.

The New Encyclopedia of Common Diseases, Rodale Press, Emmaus, Pennsylvania, 1984.

Omnibus Budget Reconcilliation Act, (OBRA), 1987.

Rider, Janice, Elizabeth Nowlis and Patricia Bentz, *Modules for Basic Nursing Skills*, Houghton Mifflin, Boston, Massachussetts, 1980.

Schniedman, Rose, Susan Lambert and Barbara Wander, *Being a Nursing Assistant*, 5th Ed., Prentice Hall, New Jersey, 1989.

Sorrentino, Sheila, *Mosby's Textbook for Nursing Assistants*, C.V. Mosby, St. Louis, Missouri, 1987.

Will, Connie and Judith Eighmy, *Being a Long-Term Care Nursing Assistant*, 2nd Ed., Prentice Hall, New Jersey, 1988.

Glossary of Terms

A

AIDS	Acquired Immune Deficiency Syndrome—disease that attacks the immune system, preventing the body from fighting infection
abduction	moving body part away from normal position
abuse	physical, mental, or sexual harm, exploitation or neglect
acetest	test to detect acetone
acidosis	inability of the body to remove toxins
adduction	moving body part toward body
alignment	keeping a straight line
apical pulse	pulse felt at the apex of the heart, under the left breast
arteriosclerosis	hardening of the arteries
arteries	blood vessels that carry blood from the heart to the system
artifact	object or possession
asepsis	free from disease producing microorganisms
aspiration	breathing in solids
assault	threat of bodily harm
assistive device	any item that helps a person regain use of a function
atherosclerosis	blockage of the arteries by deposits such as fat or cholesterol
atrophy	wasting away of muscles
attitude	the way a person acts
autoclave	intense heat sterilizing
axillary	in the armpit

B

BP cuff	instrument for measuring blood pressure
bacteria	germs causing disease and/or infection
barrier	an obstacle blocking approach
battery	physical attack or harm
bedpan	a pan used for elimination while confined to bed
bedsores	body sores caused by pressure or chafing; also called decubitus ulcers
body mechanics	proper body position to avoid injury

C

CPR	cardiopulmonary resuscitation, first-aid procedure for sudden cardiac or respiratory arrest
capillary	smallest of the blood vessels
carotid pulse	pulse found at the neck
catheter	drain tube for bladder
center of gravity	area where the bulk of an object is centered
cerebral	pertaining to the brain
cerebral vascular accident	stroke (CVA)
chemotherapy	treatment using drugs
clinitest	urine test for sugar
combustible	material that will burn
commode	moveable chair containing a built-in bedpan
confidentiality	keeping information private
constipation	difficult or painful bowel movement
consume	taking into the body
contaminate	contact with a non-sterile object
contraction	shortening and thickening of a muscle

D

decubitus ulcers	bedsores or pressure sores
defamation	oral or written words that damage someone's reputation
defecate	eliminating waste from the bowels
degenerate	breaking down
dehydration	excessive loss of water from the body
dementia	mental abilities worsen steadily
denial	refusing to believe
dentures	false teeth
depression	low spirits, sadness, dejection
diabetes	disorder of carbohydrate metabolism
diastolic pressure	lowest pressure, when the heart is relaxed
disinfection	killing or slowing the growth of most microorganisms
drawsheet	sheet used to move patient
dysphagia	difficulty swallowing

E

edema	swelling
elasticity	flexibility
elder abuse	the mistreatment of an elderly person
elimination	the process of removing wastes from the body
embolus	a blood clot carried to the brain by the circulatory system
enema	injecting fluids into the rectum
epilepsy	chronic disease of the nervous system characterized by seizures
erection	in males, when the penis becomes rigid
ethics	a standard of conduct
expiration	breathing out
extremity	a hand or foot

F

false documentation	knowingly recording incorrect information in a patient's record
feces	body waste from the bowel
feedback	checking for evidence that a message is understood
femoral pulse	pulse point in the groin (where abdomen joins thigh)
fiber	roughage essential for proper elimination
flaccid	weak and limp

G

gesture	body movements that express an idea
glucose	sugar
grand mal seizure	type of seizure resulting in the loss of consciousness
grief	reaction to loss

H

HBV	Hepatitis B virus
health-care team	personnel involved in patient care
Heimlich maneuver	first-aid procedure for choking
hemiplegia	paralysis on one side of the body
hemiparesis	loss of sensation

hemorrhage	bleeding
hygiene	cleanliness and health
HIV	Human Immunodeficiency Virus which causes AIDS
hyperglycemia	abnormally high levels of sugar in the blood
hypertension	blood pressure higher than normal
hypoglycemia	abnormally low level of sugar in the blood
hypotension	blood pressure lower than normal

I

incontinence	inability to control bladder and/or bowel functions
immune	not subject to a particular disease because of the presence of antibodies
impaction	inability to pass feces
infection	invasion of disease producing microorganisms
inspiration	breathing in
insulin	hormone produced by the pancreas which breaks down sugars and starches
insulin shock	resulting from too much insulin or too little food
intake/output	measure of fluid taken in and voided
intravenous	going directly into the vein
isolation	separating infectious patient from others

L

lethargy	abnormal drowsiness or lack of energy
lift sheet	sheet used to move patient
log rolling	method to move patient from side to side

M

Maslowe, Abraham	psychologist whose theory of the hierarchy of human needs helps explain behavior
microorganism	disease-producing bacteria seen only with a microscope
myocardial infarction	heart attack

N

NPO patients	nothing-by-mouth patients
nasogastric tube	soft plastic tube inserted through nose into stomach for feeding and/or medicating
negligence	failure to perform an act that results in injury

122

non-ambulatory	patient that cannot walk
nonverbal	unspoken communication
nutrients	substances necessary to life

O

objective reporting	stating facts
obstruction	blockage of the airway
oral	mouth
osteoporosis	bones become brittle due to calcium loss

P

pacemaker	regulates the heartbeat
pathogens	harmful germs
pedal pulse	pulse site at top front of shin
perineal	rectal and genital areas
personal hygiene	proper cleanliness and grooming
petit mal	a partial seizure which does not result in loss of consciousness
philosophy	point of view
popliteal pulse	pulse point at back of knee
prosthesis	artificial body part
psychomotor seizure	temporary loss of judgment and motor control

R

radial pulse	pulse felt at the wrist
radiation	therapy using high-energy waves
rapport	a close or sympathetic relationship
reciprocal walker	a hinged frame that moves forward one side at a time
rehabilitation	restoring a person's physical and/or mental abilities
respiration	breathing, consisting of one inspiration and one expiration
responsibility	being accountable
restraint	limits movement
rupture	the tearing apart of tissue

S

seizure	a sudden attack with convulsions
sexuality	characteristic of being male or female

shock	shut down of the cardiovascular system
slander	written statement that damages another's reputation
slide board	board used to transfer patient when there is no chance of spinal injury
spasm	involuntary muscle contractions
sphygmomanometer	measures blood pressure (also called a BP cuff)
sterile	absence of all disease-producing microorganisms
sterilization	process of killing ALL microorganisms
stethoscope	instrument used to hear sounds in the body
stroke	loss of blood to brain; also called cerebral vascular accident
stupor	a state in which the senses are partially or completely dulled
subjective reporting	reporting impressions or feelings
support	to carry or bear a specific weight
systolic pressure	highest pressure, when the heart contracts

T

temperature	measurement of body heat
therapeutic	aids good health
thermometer	instrument for measuring temperature
thrombus	a blood clot in the brain
transfer	moving from one place to another
transmit	to pass from one subject to another
trapeze bar	bar above bed to help patient move or exercise

U

universal precautions	methods to prevent infection from blood or body fluids
urinal	bedpan used by males for urinating

V

vein	blood vessel that carries blood to the heart
verbal	words (spoken or written)
vital signs	temperature, pulse, respiration, and blood pressure
void	urinate

W

wellness	absence of illness

Index

Tips and Terms Flashcards

POCKET REFERENCE—Abbreviations 1
Amounts

amt

cc

tbsp

tsp

oz

L

POCKET REFERENCE—Abbreviations 2
Activities

ADL

amb

W/C

ROM

PT

POCKET REFERENCE—Abbreviations 3
Measurements

ht

wt

lb

ft

in

POCKET REFERENCE—Abbreviations 4
Elimination

BM

BRP

U/A

S/A

spec

I/O

Measurements

- height
- weight
- pound
- feet
- inches

Elimination

- bowel movement
- bathroom privileges
- urinalysis
- sugar/acetone (urine test)
- specimen
- intake and output

Amounts

- amount
- cubic centimeter
- tablespoon
- teaspoon
- ounce
- liter

Activities

- activities of daily living
- ambulate
- wheelchair
- range of motion
- physical therapy

POCKET REFERENCE—Abbreviations 5
Body Parts

pt

abd

R

ax

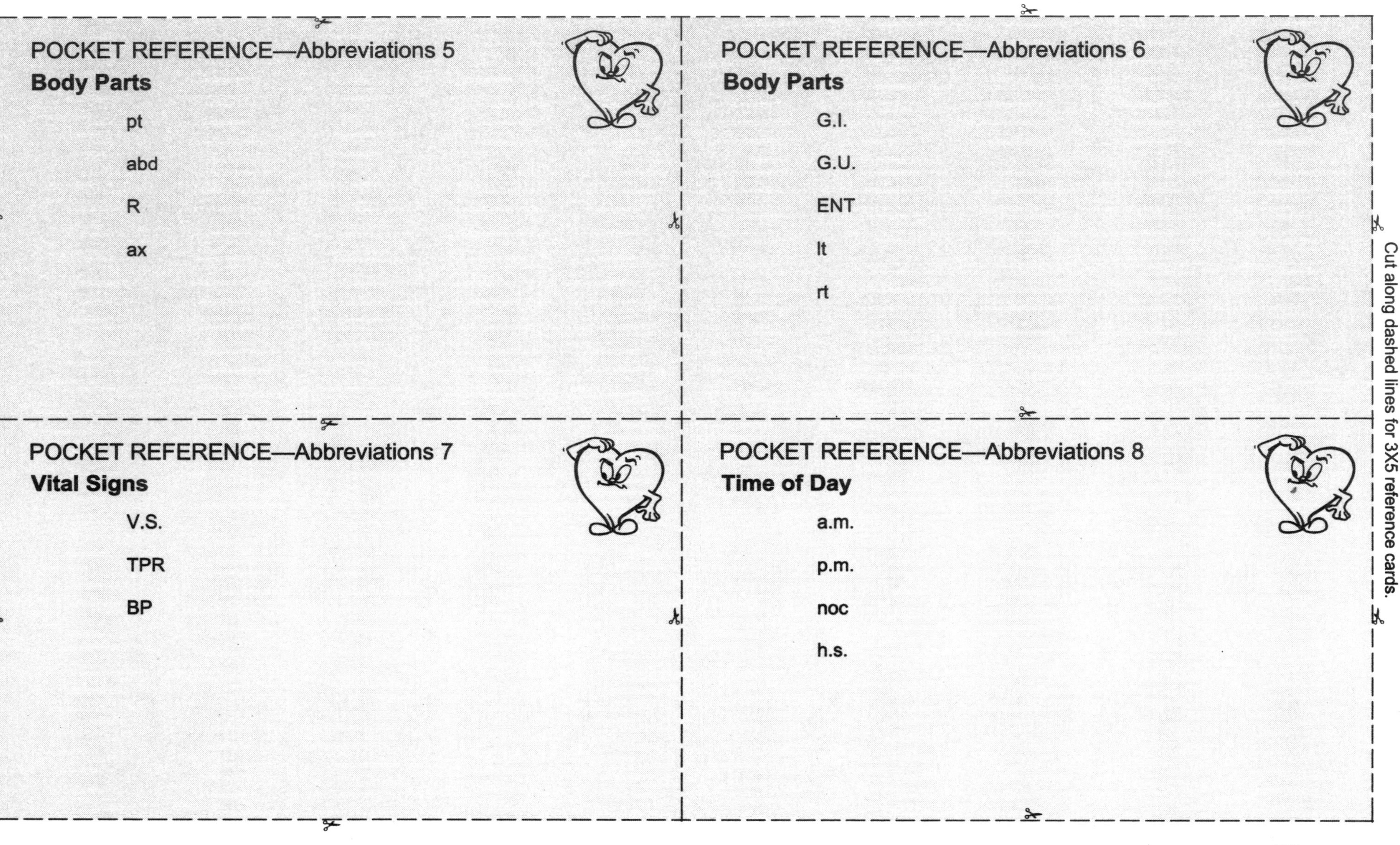

POCKET REFERENCE—Abbreviations 6
Body Parts

G.I.

G.U.

ENT

lt

rt

POCKET REFERENCE—Abbreviations 7
Vital Signs

V.S.

TPR

BP

POCKET REFERENCE—Abbreviations 8
Time of Day

a.m.

p.m.

noc

h.s.

Tips and Terms Flashcards

Vital Signs

vital signs

temperature, pulse, respiration

blood pressure

Time of Day

morning

afternoon or evening

night

bedtime (hour of sleep)

Body Parts

patient

abdomen

rectal

axillary (armpit)

Body Parts

gastrointestinal
(stomach and intestine)

genitourinary
(genital and urinary organs)

ears, nose, throat

left

right

Cut along dashed lines for 3X5 reference cards.

POCKET REFERENCE—Abbreviations 9
Time (when)

$\bar{a}$

$\bar{p}$

a.c.

p.c.

ad lib

p.r.n.

STAT

POCKET REFERENCE—Abbreviations 10
Time (frequency)

q.h.

q.d.

q.o.d.

b.i.d.

t.i.d.

q.i.d.

POCKET REFERENCE—Abbreviations 11
Medical Staff

CN

DON

RN

LPN

LVN

Dr.

POCKET REFERENCE—Abbreviations 12
Instructions

po

NPO

H_2O

$\bar{c}$

$\bar{s}$

DC

Medical Staff

charge nurse

director of nursing

registered nurse

licensed practical nurse

licensed vocational nurse

doctor

Instructions

by mouth (oral)

nothing by mouth

water

with

without

discontinue

Time (when)

before

after

before meals

after meals

as desired

as necessary

immediately

Time (frequency)

every hour

every day

every other day

two times a day

three times a day

four times a day

POCKET REFERENCE—Abbreviations 13
Treatment

Rx

IV

O_2

FF

CBR

POCKET REFERENCE—Abbreviations 14
Complications

SOB

HOH

c/o

Fx

staph

POCKET REFERENCE—Abbreviations 15
Specific Disorders

MI

CHF

CVA

Ca

AD

UTI

URI

POCKET REFERENCE—Abbreviations 16
Diagnostics

Dx

EEG

EKG or ECG

RBC

WBC

136

Specific Disorders

myocardial infarction (heart attack)

congestive heart failure

cerebral vascular accident (stroke)

cancer

Alzheimer's Disease

urinary tract infection

upper respiratory infection

Diagnostics

diagnosis

electroencephalogram (brain waves)

electrocardiogram (heart)

red blood count

white blood count

Treatment

prescription

intravenous

oxygen

force fluids

complete bed rest

Complications

shortness of breath

hard of hearing

complains of

fracture

staphylococcus (germ)

Cut along dashed lines for 3X5 reference cards.

POCKET REFERENCE—Word Parts 1
Medical Conditions

-emia   -oma

-uria   -plegia

-itis   -phasia

-stomy   -rrhage

-stasis   -rrhea

-pathy

POCKET REFERENCE—Observations 1
Pneumonia

Describe:

List symptoms:

Action to take:

POCKET REFERENCE—Observations 2
Diabetes Complications

List complications:

List symptoms for each:

Action to take:

POCKET REFERENCE—Observations 3
Alzheimer's Disease/Dementia

Describe:

List symptoms:

Action to take:

Diabetes Complications

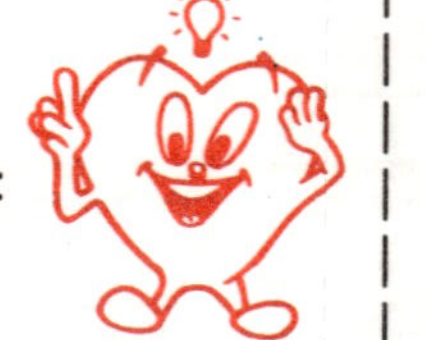

Diabetic coma symptoms:	Insulin shock symptoms:
comes on gradually	comes on suddenly
acetone breath (smells fruity)	weak, dizzy, trembling
increased urination	perspiring
thirsty	vision problems
nausea	hungry
heavy breathing	shallow respiration
flushed, hot, dry skin	pale, cold, clammy
high blood sugar	low blood sugar

Action: life-threatening; report immediately

Alzheimer's Disease/Dementia

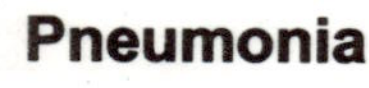

Description: progressive mental deterioration

Symptoms: unable to remember recent events
increased confusion
decreased attention span
tires easily
uncontrolled behavior
increased anxiety

Action: report and chart changes in behavior;
be patient; give simple instructions,
one step at a time; supervise closely

Medical Conditions

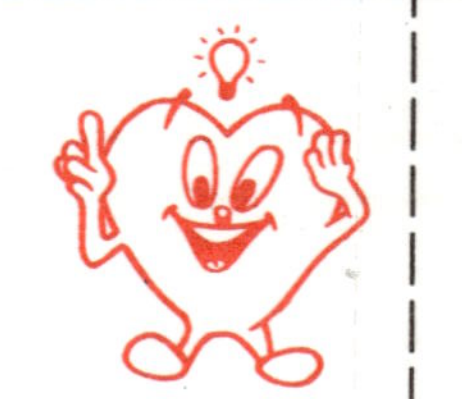

blood condition	tumor
urine condition	paralysis
inflammation	speaking
creation of an opening	excessive flow
maintaining	flow or discharge
disease	

Pneumonia

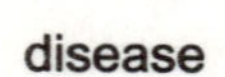

Description: acute lung disease

Symptoms: coughing
pain in chest
feverish
congested

Action: report and chart

Tips and Terms Flashcards

POCKET REFERENCE—Observations 4

Cardiac Arrest

Describe:

List symptoms:

Action to take:

POCKET REFERENCE—Observations 5

Choking

Describe:

List symptoms:

Action to take:

POCKET REFERENCE—Observations 6

Cerebral Vascular Accident (CVA)

Describe:

List Symptoms:

Action to take:

POCKET REFERENCE—Observations 7

Depression

Describe:

List symptoms:

Action to take:

Cerebral Vascular Accident (CVA)

Description: caused by blood clot or bleeding in the brain

Symptoms:
paralysis on one side
loss of sensation on one side
eyelid or mouth droops
spasms or loss of muscle control
speech problems

Actions: report and chart changes in condition; supervise carefully to protect from injury; encourage and praise independence

Depression

Description: acute sadness

Symptoms:
loss of appetite
withdrawn
low self-esteem
lack of interest or enthusiasm

Action: report and chart changes; express concern and interest; take time to talk (but don't force conversation); motivate to participate in activities; help to feel good about self and appearance

Cardiac Arrest

Description: the heart stops pumping

Symptoms:
no chest movement
no breath, or breathing is extremely difficult
unconscious
skin, lips, and nails turn blue-gray

Action: life-threatening; call for help immediately; begin CPR

Choking

Description: obstructed airway

Symptoms:
clutching the throat
unable to breathe
cannot speak or cough

Action: life-threatening; call for help immediately; begin the Heimlich Maneuver

Cut along dashed lines for 3X5 reference cards.

POCKET REFERENCE—Observations 8
Urinary Infection

Describe:

List symptoms:

List some causes:

Action to take:

POCKET REFERENCE—Observations 9
Allergic Reaction

Describe:

List symptoms:

Action to take:

POCKET REFERENCE—Observations 10
Myocardial Infarction (MI)

Describe:

List symptoms:

Action to take:

POCKET REFERENCE—Observations 11
Congestive Heart Failure

Describe:

List symptoms:

Action to take:

Myocardial Infarction (MI)

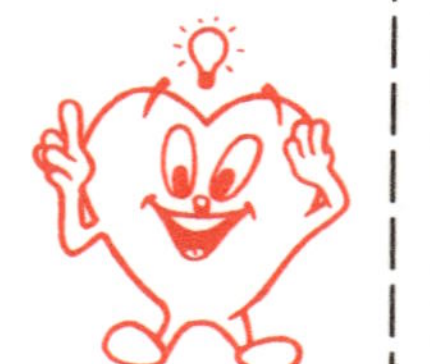

Description: heart attack

Symptoms: chest pain
pale, cold, clammy
pain in left arm and neck
irregular, weak pulse
decreased blood pressure

Action: life-threatening; report immediately

Congestive Heart Failure

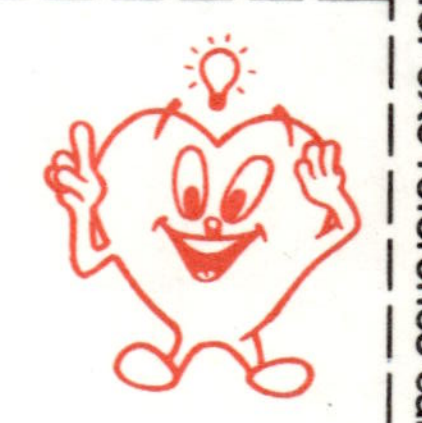

Description: circulatory congestion
caused by heart disorders

Symptoms: lung congestion
chest discomfort
swelling in extremities
weight gain
restlessness
breathing difficulty
dizzy, confused, tired

Action: emergency situation; report
immediately

Urinary Infection

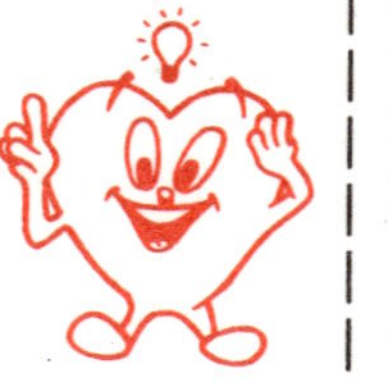

Description: infection of the urinary system

Symptoms: pain in lower back
pain or burning with urination
change in urine odor, color, frequency

Some causes: insufficient fluids
poor perineal care
unable to empty bladder completely
indwelling catheter
bedridden/inactivity

Action: report and chart; encourage fluids

Allergic Reaction

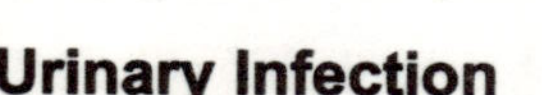

Description: sensitivity to specific foods
or medications

Symptoms: itching or tingling
skin rashes
rapid swelling
breathing difficulty
vision problems
scratchy throat

Action: emergency situation; report immediately

Tips and Terms Flashcards

POCKET REFERENCE—Observations 12

Edema

Describe:

List symptoms:

Action to take:

POCKET REFERENCE—Observations 13

Dehydration

Describe:

List symptoms:

Action to take:

POCKET REFERENCE—Observations 14

Approaching Death

Describe:

List symptoms:

Action to take:

POCKET REFERENCE—Observations 15

Decubitus Ulcer

Describe:

Cause:

List symptoms:

Action to take:

Approaching Death

Description: final stages of life

Symptoms:
cold hands and feet
blank stare
pale or gray
perspiring
limp
slow or difficult breathing
rattling sound in throat or chest
rapid, weak pulse

Actions: report immediately; continue giving the best care possible; keep the room well ventilated and lighted; offer comfort and support to the patient and the family; provide privacy with loved ones

Decubitus Ulcer

Description: bed sore or pressure sore

Cause: pressure on body parts that are not protected by fatty tissues; shoulder blades, elbows, toes, feet, etc.

Symptoms: redness that does not disappear when pressure is relieved

area is tender and warmer than other skin
blisters or open sores that can lead to infection

Action: keep skin clean and dry; massage gently; keep bed free of wrinkles; encourage fluids; reposition frequently; follow the facility's procedures for cushioning or bridging; report and chart

Edema

Description: fluid retention

Symptoms:
swollen feet, ankles, face,
fingers, joints, tissues
weight gain
decreased urine output

Action: report and chart changes; elevate swollen area; encourage loose-fitting clothing

Dehydration

Description: lack of fluids

Symptoms:
excessive thirst
decreased urine output
constipation
dry skin, lips, tongue
decreased blood pressure
rapid, weak pulse

Action: affect all body systems and can be life-threatening; report immediately